The Practice Manager

THIRD EDITION

Edited by

Michael Drury

AND

Lynne Hobden-Clarke

Provided as an educational service by

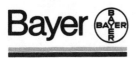

RADCLIFFE MEDICAL PRESS
OXFORD and NEW YORK

© 1994 Radcliffe Medical Press Ltd
15 Kings Meadow, Ferry Hinksey Road, Oxford OX2 0DP

141 Fifth Avenue, New York, NY 10010, USA

First Edition 1990
Reprinted 1990
Reprinted 1991
Second Edition 1991
Reprinted 1992
Reprinted 1993
Third Edition 1994
Reprinted 1995

British Library Cataloguing in Publication Data

A catalogue record is available from the British Library

ISBN 1 85775 050 0

Typeset by AMA Graphics Ltd, Preston
Printed and bound in Great Britain by
Biddles Ltd, Guildford and King's Lynn

Contents

Preface to the First Edition

THIS book is written for the practice managers and senior receptionists. Whilst it will stand on its own, it is designed to accompany Practice Manager Development, a course in which a group of practice managers (and sometimes doctors) learn together and from each other. Whilst nearly all group practices now have a practice manager their experience and skills are very varied. Some, probably the majority, have been promoted within the practice from receptionist and have learnt and developed as time has passed. These have very often had little opportunity to learn outside the practice, little chance to get support and education from their peer group and it has been difficult to introduce modern management skills from different business areas. A few have come from outside with previous management training but have had to learn the medical component of their job the hard way. This book is designed primarily for the former group but we hope that any practice manager would be helped by it.

The authors have been drawn from outside disciplines and from the medical world in an attempt to get the balance right; the book therefore covers both concepts and practical issues. Managers are concerned with people, equipment and money and the management of all these aspects of general practice is considered.

Not all practice managers are female but for the sake of continuity we have written as if they are and as if the doctors are male. We hope this device will not offend others.

We are grateful to Drs Fleming, Oldroyd, Ridsdill-Smith, Taylor, Pike and Steel who, sometimes with their practice managers, advised on the content of the book. We are also grateful to a large number of secretaries who have helped. Finally, our thanks go to Andrew Bax and Kate Martin at Radcliffe Medical Press and to Ciba-Geigy Pharmaceuticals whose financial help made publication possible.

Professor Sir Michael Drury
Department of General Practice
University of Birmingham

November 1989

Preface to the Second Edition

THE wide acceptance of the first edition of this book has been responsible for the need to reprint it during its first year. Further demand has given an opportunity to produce a Second Edition and to add some new sections, keeping it thoroughly up to date with the rapid changes in the health service. In particular, sections have been added to cover audit, practice prescribing budgets and fund holding. We have also taken the opportunity to make alterations to those sections covering communication, motivation and team-work as well as revising most other chapters. All concerned in this new edition recognize the importance of the role of practice managers in today's health service and hope that this book will help them with their tasks and add to the satisfaction they obtain.

I would like to acknowledge the help of David Clegg and Michael Hamilton, who have joined our team of contributors for this edition, and of Janice Downing and Pauline Shepherd, who advised in its preparation.

Professor Sir Michael Drury
Department of General Practice
University of Birmingham

May 1991

Preface to the Third Edition

Despite the popularity of the first two editions of this book the rapidity of change in general practice has meant that a third edition is required, only four years after its first appearance, to ensure that it is thoroughly up-to-date.

We have made radical changes, including enlisting more practice managers as contributors, who now provide almost half the content, and sharing the task of editing. Computing now merits a separate chapter and the chapter on fundholding has been revised and expanded. Issues of quality are dealt with in the sections on audit and in the final chapter.

We are grateful for the enthusiastic support of contributing authors and to the editorial staff at Radcliffe Medical Press. Finally, we are aware that the pace of change is unlikely to slacken and would therefore welcome any suggestions from our readers on how this book may be further improved.

Sir Michael Drury,
Emeritus Professor of General Practice,
University of Birmingham

Mrs Lynne Hobden-Clarke,
Practice Manager,
Gerrards Cross

Publisher's Note

Gender is an issue which always provokes controversy and comment, and there is no successful formula which can avoid it. Readers of this book will notice that some chapters are written as if all practice managers are female, and others as if they are male. Although it would normally be part of our editorial process to make the text consistent in such matters, we decided, on this occasion, to leave it according to the contributors' style. This policy will not satisfy the purists, and to them we can only apologize.

However, all of us know that practice managers can be of either sex, and we ask those who use this book to read it with this reality in mind.

Radcliffe Medical Press
July 1994

List of Authors

Bernard Baillon
General Practitioner, Northampton; Associate Adviser,
Oxford Regional Health Authority

Sue Casement
Practice Manager, Maidenhead

John Dean
Director, John Dean Associates; formerly Director of Medical Services,
Pannell Kerr Forster

Sir Michael Drury
Past President of the Royal College of General Practitioners

Norman Ellis
Under Secretary, British Medical Association

Lynne Hobden-Clarke
Practice Manager, Chalfont St Peter; Editorial Adviser,
Practice Manager

Roderick Martin
Professor of Organizational Behaviour and Director of Glasgow
University Business School, Glasgow

Angela Scott
Practice Manager, Leighton Buzzard

Paula Taft
Practice Manager, Birmingham

Christopher Trower
Medical Director, Buckinghamshire Family Health Services Authority

Richard Wilkinson
General Practitioner, Bremsgrove

1 The Nature of General Practice

THIS chapter aims to explore the philosophy of general practice. What are its objectives? What is the nature of the problems that it faces and what solutions does it offer? These questions are important ones for the practice manager to address because she will have to subscribe to that philosophy if she is to make the most of her contribution to patient care.

Everyone who considers himself or herself to be ill needs a point of first contact with a physician which allows entry into the health care system. This frontline medical care is known as 'primary care' in contrast to that of 'secondary care' which is specialized and more sophisticated than that handled in primary care and to which access is usually gained only after being filtered or sorted within primary care. Most countries have some such system but whereas in the UK it is called 'general practice' in other countries it may be 'family practice', 'primary medical care' or 'primary health care'. Whatever the title it has certain characteristics above and beyond being a point of first contact.

1 *The problem presented is undifferentiated.* People do not have to make decisions about the nature of their problem, only that they have one and that it is probably concerned with their health. They do not have to decide whether their chest pain is due to their heart, in which case they would need the advice of a cardiologist or that it may be indigestion and a stomach specialist would be more appropriate. Their problems may be life-threatening or they may be trivial. Furthermore it is the patient's perception of this which is relevant, not the receptionist's, the manager's or the doctor's, so access to care has to be as unrestricted as possible. This is a very important idea to grasp because it clearly shapes how we behave to patients, what we say and the sort of systems that we organize. General practice has to be 'comprehensive'.

2 *Care is offered to the family group.* The fact that problems are undifferentiated and that any age may attend obviously allows all members of the family to be seen but the concept embraced is wider than this. All illness should be regarded as potentially 'family illness'. It is clear that, say, marital disharmony will affect the husband and wife and almost certainly have an impact on children, grandparents and even brothers and sisters whose

affections can be stressed. It is not so obvious that, say, a duodenal ulcer can affect the family but the diet, the need for rest and quiet, the effect upon temper, holidays, sexual relationships can all be factors in the management. Another perspective of the significance of family care is the need to explore and make the best of this opportunity within a consultation. The spouse who accompanies the patient is expressing concern and caring and needs to be considered. The act of immunizing a child is more than giving an injection, it is an opportunity to establish a relationship with a mother, to discuss feeding, growth, education and behaviour at a time when the mother is very receptive to these ideas.

3 *Care is continuous.*   Much care is episodic. A patient may come once with a boil, take advice, perhaps receive a prescription and have urine tested for glycosuria and then leave, but most care is prolonged for most illness is chronic or recurrent. Tables 1.1, 1.2 and 1.3 show the approximate frequency with which common and rare problems may be seen in a practice of 10 000 persons and it will be noted that chronic disease is a longer list and represents several consultations for that condition each year. The right-hand figure gives the number of persons consulting per year from a list of 10 000 patients.

Nearly all chronic disease is now treated within the community. Some, such as hypertension, are nearly always treated within general practice, but

Table 1.1   Minor conditions.

	No. of cases per year/10 000 patients
Tonsillitis	400
Acute otitis media	350
Cystitis	200
Back pain	200
Migraine	120
Hay fever	100

Table 1.2   Acute major conditions.

	No. of cases per year/10 000 patients
Acute chest infection	200
Coronary thomboses	30
Acute appendix	20
Stroke	20
All cancers	20

Table 1.3 Some chronic disease in general practice: annual person consulting rates.

	Annual persons consulting per 10 000 patients
High blood pressure	1000
Chronic rheumatism, arthritis	400
Chronic mental	400
Ischaemic heart disease	200
Obesity	200
All cancers	120
Asthma	120
Diabetes	120
Strokes	80
Epilepsy	40
Multiple sclerosis	12

From: *N.H.S. Data Book*, eds Fry, J., Brooks, D. & McColl, I.M.T. Press Ltd. (1984).

other problems may sometimes be treated by other agencies, specialists, hospitals, private sources and so on. However, because primary care is continuous the record card is the only repository of all medical information and the responsibility for manipulating and co-ordinating care across boundaries, in short 'managing', is the task of general practice. That is why we have a referral system and why all the letters eventually return from the periphery to the centre of the web. The patient with a stroke may be seen at the hospital, or even admitted for a while, but the responsibility for continuity of care, for organizing transport, meals-on-wheels, physiotherapy or chiropody is ultimately that of general practice although, of course, it is often convenient to delegate it to others. Again the implications of this concept are great and the practice team has a vital role in co-ordinating good quality care. Certainly patients see this as a most important function and its breakdown as a fearful addition to existing problems of ill health.

It also has very important implications for management in terms of activity. Letters arrive from hospitals asking us to prescribe a drug, arrange an investigation or review after a period of time and that action has to be taken otherwise the patient may suffer, the hospital be given extra work or even litigation ensue.

Continuity of care has one other aspect that must be considered here. Care given by a variety of people can soon become fragmented and confusing for the patient. It needs some skill directed to the problem to enable one person, or as few people as necessary to become involved. For example a patient dying at home needs to be cared for by their nurse and their doctor. At the same time cover by other informed people is necessary when the key people cannot be there.

4 *Care includes disease prevention and health promotion.*   One of the most profound shifts in the philosophy of general practice in the past few years has been the change from a 'reactive' pattern of working to a 'pro-active' one. The best simile is that provided by the fire brigade. Their 'reactive' pattern of work is to sally forth at high speed in response to a call that your house is on fire. Their 'pro-active' work involves calling to advise on safety precautions, fire-proof doors, smoke detectors, etc. that might prevent a catastrophe. Similarly, in general practice, when a family registers with the practice they are saying 'please be there when we want you' but they are also saying 'please stop us suffering from illness that can be avoided'. Of course patients are autonomous; they are at liberty to decline, without fear of causing offence, the advice that is offered, but it is the responsibility of the health professional to make certain that they are informed, and understand the issues. A general practice has a responsibility for each individual patient but it has also a wider responsibility to its whole population. We need to protect from infectious disease by immunizing the well; to detect early illness by measuring blood pressure, screening for cancer of the cervix or high blood cholesterol and to promote good health by considering diet, smoking, alcohol intake, exercise and relaxation in well people.

Why us and not someone else you may ask? We have two great assets on our side. Firstly most people see a doctor regularly. Every year nearly 70% of the people on our list will attend the surgery; by the end of two years that figure will have risen to 80% and by a further year to 90%. That provides a tremendous chance for opportunistic screening or advice giving, but if it is to be effective every person in the team needs to be alert to that chance. Secondly patients are 'switched on' to health concerns when they consult so health education makes a great impact at this time. Fear is a great force towards taking action to prevent ill health.

5 *Care attends to the whole person.*   Wholism has become something of a cliché in the past few years and the concept has been grasped by others who have often accused the medical profession of being so disease-centred – 'he was only interested in my liver' – that they ignored the person outside the disease. There is some justification in this view in some of our behaviour but we have moved progressively further towards a much more rounded ap-proach. We are now comfortable with this and have encapsulated the concept by constructing diagnoses or management plans in interlocking areas of physical, psychological and social factors.

Clearly at times, or with particular diseases one of these components is predominant. A young man with a fractured tibia has a largely physical problem, but even here there may be anxiety about his ability to play football

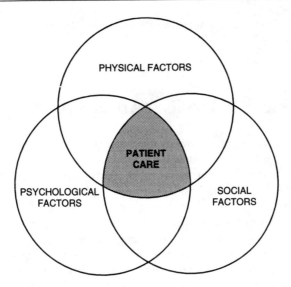

Figure 1.1:   The factors affecting patient care.

in the future that constitutes a major worry and problems with his work of a social nature. If these are not considered he may rightly feel incompletely cared for. In other situations, such as malignant disease or depression other areas become predominant but they are all always there. Administration needs to grasp this idea if it is to recognize the different reasons for seeking care and the different patterns of behaviour of those who come.

In 1969 the Royal College of General Practitioners published a job definition of the general practitioner and it is as true today as when it was first written.

Job definition

'The general practitioner is a doctor who provides personal, primary and continuing medical care to individuals and families. He may attend his patients in their homes, in his consulting-room or sometimes in hospital. He accepts the responsibility for making an initial decision on every problem his patient may present to him, consulting with specialists when he thinks it appropriate to do so. He will usually work in a group with other general practitioners, from premises that are built or modified for the purpose, with the help of paramedical colleagues, adequate secretarial staff and all the equipment which is necessary. Even if he is in single-handed practice, he will work in a team and delegate when necessary. His diagnoses will be composed in physical, psychological and social terms. He will intervene educationally, preventively and therapeutically to promote his patient's health.'

(From p.1 of *The Future General Practitioner*, Royal College of General Practitioners, 1972.)

Family Health Services Authority

Most practice managers will already have a clear understanding of the structure of the practice within which they work so this chapter will not describe this but will concentrate, rather, on the ideas behind the structure and the way it is changing and will seek to explore some of the philosophy behind these changes. We shall describe briefly some of the outside organizations with which general practice relates as the new functions and structure of these may be less well-known to practice managers.

The general practitioner (GP) has a different relationship with the health service to that of doctors working in hospitals. He is not an employee of the health service as they are but an independent contractor. This is an important difference which shapes and directs the way in which general practice is managed and develops. To understand the concept of 'independent contractor status' it is helpful to use an analogy from the construction industry. The builder who has the task of developing a housing estate directly employs a number of workers who labour, lay bricks and work with timber. He also needs electricity put into these houses – wiring, plugs, cooker points and so on – but he does not directly employ electricians so he gives a contract to a firm of electricians to do this, specifying what is required and how much he will pay for the completed job but he leaves the details of the work to the 'independent' firm to arrange and only requires a satisfactory job to be done within the time and price agreed by the firm who is thus an 'independent contractor'. In this same way the GP has a contract to supply services to patients who are registered by the Family Health Services Authority (FHSA) as on his list. It is his responsibility to provide the premises, time, equipment and systems required to do a proper job. There is considerable flexibility about how and where he does this providing that it is done within the broad guidelines of the contract.

An independent contractor is therefore a self-employed person who has entered into a contract for services with another party. This contract *for* services is fundamentally different from a contract *of* services, which governs employee–employer relationships and is explained in greater detail in *Making Sense of the New Contract* ed. J. Chisholm, Radcliffe Medical Press, Oxford (1990), but it is essentially a difference in the amount of control that exists.

The GP then is not an employee of the FHSA. If he makes a mistake the responsibility is his, not that of the FHSA. If he had been an employee then the employer, the FHSA, would also have been responsible if a mistake was made. Of course the contract agreed between the two parties is much more explicit than this and contains rules about hours of work and access by patients, about the standards of premises and where doctors may live, but much of the work is bound by general statements, such as 'a doctor shall render his patients all necessary and appropriate personal services of the type usually provided by general practitioners', or 'shall keep adequate records of the illnesses and treatment of his patient on forms supplied to him for the purpose by the Authority', or 'shall do so at his premises or, if the condition of the patient so requires, elsewhere in his practice area', etc. It will be noted at once that the use of words and phrases such as 'necessary and appropriate', 'adequate' and so on raise issues of what is adequate or necessary and by whom it is so judged.

The functions of the previous Family Practitioner Committee was mainly to administer the contract with doctors (and dentists, opticians and pharmacists) and to maintain the register of patients, and it had nearly half of its members drawn from professional bodies. With the new FHSAs this has changed. Why has this change been proposed? The answer lies partly within the concept of the independent contractor. The advantage of this system is, primarily, its flexibility. As practices can control their own methods and systems for providing care a good deal of variation occurs depending on local differences. Populations, patients, staff, buildings and local geography are all different and what suits one practice may not suit others. The potential disadvantage is that the variation may become too great. There may be such a variation that unacceptable standards are allowed to exist. The FHSA has the responsibilities of planning, developing and managing the services provided by general medical practitioners, general dental practitioners, retail pharmacists and opticians. In England there are 90 FHSAs relating to 14 Regional Health Authorities (RHAs). The eight FHSAs in Wales relate to the Welsh Office, whereas in Scotland there are 15 Health Boards responsible for hospital, community and family health services and in Northern Ireland a Central Services Agency.

The FHSAs in England look after populations ranging between 130 000 and 1 600 000. Nearly 40 of these share a boundary with a single District Health Authority (DHA) but the remainder relate to between two and seven DHAs. Each FHSA consists of a Chairman, usually a lay person, appointed by the Secretary of State, and 10 other members appointed by the Regional Health Authority; five lay people, the General Manager, a GP, a dentist, a pharmacist and a nurse. The Vice-Chairman is elected by the members.

Most FHSAs are organized around the structure of a patient data department, a finance department and a management or service development department. Other departments are involved in tasks such as dealing with stores and so on.

The patient data department relies on the individual practice for information and, as well as maintaining the register, runs the recall systems for cervical cytology and mammography.

The service development department is the area that most marks the change from administration to managing the service, and is involved in planning and strategic development. It is the department most involved with the social services department of the local authority and the District Health Authority and the Care in the Community programmes (effective from 1 April 1993). There is now to be a move towards merging FHSAs and DHAs into single authorities.

In England the FHSA is accountable to the Regional Health Authority. The functions of the FHSA, in relationship to general practice, are to:

- manage the contracts of GPs;
- pay GPs;
- provide information to the public;
- deal with complaints made by patients;
- assess the health needs of the population;
- develop services that are effective and efficient.

The last two of these functions are relatively new but in spite of these additions general practice remains the least 'organized' part of the National Health Service with very little direct local management accountability for the services delivered or the resources consumed.

There are major forces for change (*see* Figure 1.2), many of which are already impinging on the tasks of practice managers. There is a great pressure to devolve some care from secondary services to primary care. This is manifested particularly by the shifts in care of patients with chronic illness or minor illness to general practice, in areas of prescribing and in the move of diagnostic services closer to the patient.

The Community Care Act (1990) marks another aspect of this shift, with its intention to promote the development of services to enable people to live in their homes wherever feasible. The responsibility for this has now been

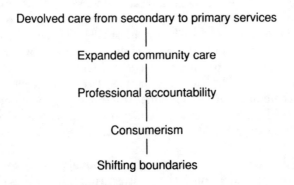

Devolved care from secondary to primary services

Expanded community care

Professional accountability

Consumerism

Shifting boundaries

Figure 1.2:   Forces for change in primary care.

moved to local authorities and we do not yet know how much the tasks of assessment and expanded care will impinge on general practice.

There is an increased element of consumerism, which is referred to elsewhere in the book, that expects a response from primary care and will change both attitudes and behaviour. Bound up with this is the general trend, to be found in every public service, for more accountability leading to better management of resources.

Lastly, are the factors stemming from the changes in the 1990 contract – medical audit, the impact of fundholding, and the shifting boundaries between hospital doctors and general practitioners, between nurses and doctors, between the statutory services and voluntary services and between private and state medicine.

In spite of all these pressures for change, we have to remember that it is the consultation between doctor and patient, in the assured privacy of the consulting room, that remains at the heart of our task.

2 The Nature of Management and Administration

Introduction

GENERAL practice managers are unique. The majority of managers—there were over 2 1/2 million of them in 1988—work in a specific function within a large organization, either in the private or the public sector. They may be working in departments of finance, personnel, research and development, production, marketing and distribution, sales or after-sales service. They will be responsible for one particular aspect of their firm's work. For example, an individual personnel manager may be responsible for the pay and conditions of non-manual staff. Here, they will be directly responsible to a more senior manager, the departmental head, and through him to more senior managers (there are characteristically seven levels of managers in a large organization, although there may be as many as 12). In addition, the individual manager may have a 'dotted line' relationship with yet another senior manager. For example, the plant personnel manager is responsible on a day-to-day basis to the plant director, and to the senior personnel director at head office for overall policy.

The general practice manager works in a quite different setting. She is part of a large public sector organization, the National Health Service, which is the largest employer in Europe. However, she will work in a relatively small organization, with perhaps up to ten staff. The number of practices with five or more partners is increasing, and such practices may have as many as 40 staff in total, but such large practices are not the most common. It is estimated that only 10 000 of Britain's 32 000 GPs work in practices with four or more partners. Unlike most managers, the practice manager will have a much wider range of responsibilities: for people, for money, for office procedures, for relations with patients, for relations with other medical agencies, and for dealing with the general public. She will not be helped, and protected, by a large staff of assistants. She may have clearly defined responsibilities, set out in a detailed job description, but more likely she will not. She may have a managing partner to report to, but it is more likely that she will be equally responsible to all partners, all of whom have other major interests and responsibilities. She may have a number of assistants who handle a limited range of management responsibilities, for example finance, but again it is more likely that she will not.

The practice manager is therefore a special kind of manager, working in a small unit, with wide responsibilities and in direct contact with the general public. Her work is especially challenging, and especially visible.

The practice manager is special, but she remains a manager, with normal management responsibilities and tasks. The essence of management lies in establishing objectives, translating objectives into roles, tasks and procedures, establishing priorities, and ensuring that the objectives are achieved. This involves dealing with a wide range of people and issues, and establishing priorities between them. It involves ensuring that decisions are not ignored, or changed without thought the following month. Inside the practice the practice manager, like all managers, has to look upwards to the partners, sideways to the other practice managers and downwards to other employees of the practice. She also has to look outside the organization, to patients, to other parts of the Health Service, and to the surrounding community.

The rest of this chapter explains these general matters more fully and covers seven elements.

1 Establishing objectives.
2 Defining roles, tasks and procedures.
3 Establishing priorities.
4 Securing and allocating resources.
5 Securing compliance.
6 Monitoring performance.
7 Watching the outside world.

Establishing objectives

The specific objectives of practices may vary, and there may be differences between partners in the same practice. However, it is important that the practice should have objectives discussed and if possible agreed among the partners. This is especially important if the practice is considering the selection of a new partner, or is engaged in continuing education. Among the questions which need to be asked are: Who should define the objectives? What are the objectives and how precisely should they be defined? How often should they be reviewed? How important is it to be able to measure performance against the objectives? Should the objectives be stated in financial terms? What other measurements are appropriate?

Who should define the objectives? There is a difference between the aims of a practice and the objectives of a practice, although the two words are often used to mean the same thing. The aims of the practice may be very general to promote good health and prevent disease whenever possible. The partners are directly responsible for establishing such overall aims for the practice just as the Board of Directors is responsible for establishing the aims of a public corporation. It is not the responsibility of the practice manager to say what the aims should be, although she might have to ensure that some explicit aims exist, such as that tetanus immunization should be offered to all patients every ten years, and are discussed from time to time. But it is the responsibility of the practice manager to translate overall aims into more specific objectives, and to secure agreement from the partners that the objectives are a satisfactory method for meeting the practice's aims.

Corporation directors may define the aims of the corporation as being 'to provide technological leadership for the industry' (first of the pack) or to be at the forefront in terms of 'quality of service' (as the Lex company, which operates in leasing, has done). This is translated into the objective of being able to respond to all requests for service within a given time period. Medical practices are not public corporations, concerned with profits and market share, but they require an idea of how to translate good health care into practical terms, and to assess whether they are being successful or not. The practical measure of good health care might be reviewing all diabetic patients at agreed intervals, or limiting the delays between patients telephoning for an appointment and seeing the doctor. If possible, the objectives should be measurable by making use of information which the practice would require for other reasons, rather than establishing special requirements.

Once established, the aims of the practice should only be reviewed at long intervals. However, the objectives might be appropriately reviewed on a bi-annual basis, depending upon the frequency of changes in the practice's environment. Reviewing the objectives too frequently can be wasteful, especially if little has changed for the practice.

Business organizations typically establish a target rate of return on assets, and may establish a target market share. Practice managers will find it difficult to follow established business practice, since they are not operating in a market. However, it may be helpful to establish financial targets. If targets are established they should not be established solely in terms of costs, but in terms of returns on assets; otherwise there is the danger of being totally preoccupied with reductions in costs rather than the realization of benefits. For example, the purchase of a new ECG machine might be assessed by the use to which it is put.

Defining roles, tasks and procedures

The precise distribution of work within the practice will depend upon several factors, especially the size of the practice, the number and qualifications of the staff, the physical arrangements of the surgery, waiting room, reception area and office, and many other things. The larger the practice, and the larger the staff, the greater the importance of having clearly defined roles, tasks and procedures. However, as practices are very busy, and even practices with a few partners may have large numbers of part-time staff, it is important for matters to be defined clearly. It is especially important for the roles, tasks and procedures to be documented as there is likely to be significant turnover of staff, perhaps including turnover in practice managers.

There are three general questions.

Who is to define roles, tasks and procedures?
How closely should they be defined?
What considerations need to be taken into account when establishing the structure?

It is the practice manager's job to define the roles, tasks and procedures within the practice, except where there are clear medical issues involved. The practice manager should be familiar with the requirements of good practice management, which involves a knowledge of general office practice as well as specific features of general practice. The partners should be informed and consulted, but there is no reason to expect that GPs should be experts in management (any more than practice managers need medical qualifications). It may be helpful in group practices if one of the partners fulfils the function of the managing partner in an accountancy practice, but this role is not necessarily one which must be filled by the senior partner. It might also be helpful if one partner takes on, say, financial aspects, another education and so on but defined lines of communication should exist to avoid confusion.

Some business organizations are structured like a machine, with everything clearly defined; other business organizations operate on more 'organic' principles, with members of staff assuming a wide range of responsibilities, without clear definition. The first type of system works best when it is possible to predict what will happen perhaps because the firm is making a simple product for a known market (like bread); the second type of organization works best when circumstances are frequently changing, perhaps because of changes in technology or because the market is unpredictable (like high fashion clothing). Patients' symptoms are varied, and the job of the GP is not programmed. However, the organization of the practice can be programmed, as patients are dealt with in standard portions of time. The roles and tasks of members of staff, and the procedures to be followed, can therefore be relatively programmed and worked out on a clearly defined basis. This is particularly necessary where staff are relatively inexperienced or are working on a part-time basis and do not have the opportunity to familiarize themselves fully with the procedures followed in the surgery. There are good legal reasons as well why care protocols should be explicit for staff.

The interests of the employee as well as the interests of the partners and the patients should be taken into account when establishing patterns of work. This is especially important where the practice manager needs employees to adopt a flexible attitude towards their work, for example over standing in for other staff who are off sick or with family difficulties and when it is difficult to predict when work in an evening will end. If staff interests are ignored it is difficult to expect them to adopt a flexible attitude. The final responsibility rests with the practice manager, but she should take a wide range of interests into account and motivation becomes very important.

In many organizations the general public is invisible, or only dealt with by a small number of employees. However, in general practice the public, as patients, is centrally involved, and the practice employees are in the public eye at a time when the patient has a high level of anxiety. It is therefore necessary to pay attention to 'patient management' as well as to 'staff management' when deciding on the allocation of roles and tasks; front office as well as back office skills are required. This makes a flexible approach even more necessary.

Establishing priorities

Practice managers will always find themselves with too much to do and too little time to do it. Their staff will find the same problem. It is the practice manager's job to establish priorities, both for herself and for other members of staff. The manager's job falls into four broad types of activity; (a) report preparation; (b) internal communication; (c) external communication; and (d) meetings. The manager's work is fragmented, and only a relatively small amount of time is spent thinking or planning, or on the preparation of reports, even in large organizations. This is likely to be even more true in small organizations. However, it is important for the practice manager to avoid spending all the time dealing with yesterday's crisis, and working in a fragmented way. Spending time establishing priorities should reduce the amount of time which has to be spent in responding to yesterday's crisis. The practice manager will also need to balance pressures coming from different quarters—from doctors, other staff, patients, administrators, officials and doctors in other medical institutions. The highest immediate priority might not always be the priority established by the partners.

The specific priorities of the practice manager will vary between practices. Some practices will have a different range of issues to deal with than others, perhaps because of the clinical facilities available in the particular catchment area in which the practice is located. The establishment of medical priorities is the responsibility of the practice partners. However, the medical priorities chosen all have financial and organizational consequences and it is the job of the practice manager to establish what these are and to make them clear to the partners. There is usually a range of activities necessary for supporting the medical activities of the practice which will be primarily the responsibility of the practice manager and she is directly responsible for establishing priorities in this area.

In business organizations it is possible to establish priorities on the basis of financial criteria such as reductions in the costs of production or contributions to an increase in sales. There are some equivalents in medical practices. The costs of running the practice (staff, equipment, property costs) can be assessed and compared with the costs of other practices. It is possible to assess the effectiveness of the practice in ensuring that fees and reimbursements from the FHSA are maximized. It is, of course, also possible to assess the performance of the practice with private patients in directly economic terms.

It is particularly important to have clearly established priorities when recruiting new staff, or when investing in new equipment. When appointing new staff there is an obvious practice of simply replacing the person who has left. However, vacancies provide an opportunity to assess the overall position of the practice, and to consider whether the staffing requirements have changed since the last appointment was made. Could the work of existing staff be rearranged, either to reduce the time taken by different tasks, or to broaden the experience of existing staff? This may be a good way of making the work more interesting, as well as making it easier to cover for other staff during absences. If new staff are appointed, it might be desirable to appoint a different type of person from the person who left, perhaps to change the age distribution of staff or to introduce new skills.

The same policy of reconsidering the total picture should be adopted when buying major new pieces of equipment. In particular, the increased sophistication and reduced cost of computers has made it possible to record and store information in more efficient ways than in the past. It is possible to combine functions which had previously to be done by different people. Computerizing the practice office may be inappropriate, because it is too expensive, or because it requires too highly skilled staff, or because the working conditions in the office are too confusing for the staff to cope with the complex equipment. However, it may be that substantial improvements in efficiency are possible and as practices become more involved in the care of groups of patients, hypertensives, diabetics, asthmatics, the elderly, immunization or paediatric surveillance for example, it may become essential. The important point is not to establish an electronic office in inappropriate circumstances, but to ensure that equipment purchases are looked at in the overall context of practice requirements, for the present and the future, and not undertaken on a simple replacement basis. If the practice manger does not consider such issues, no-one else is likely to.

Hiring new staff and buying new equipment are activities common to many types of managers. But the practice manager has the difficult task of ensuring that changes which improve business efficiency do not damage patient satisfaction. The practice manager has to establish priorities where the overall objectives may not be clear-cut. In particular, medical and financial requirements have to be reconciled. It is therefore more important for the practice manager than for anyone else that the objectives of the practice should be clear, for without such guidance her job becomes impossible.

The basis for establishing priorities in business organizations is usually provided by the budget. The budget is conventionally divided into capital and operating expenditures. The practice manager has to establish priorities within the framework of the practice budget.

Securing and allocating resources

The practice manager is responsible for the preparation of the annual budget and for securing fees and reimbursements from the FHSA. The practice manager should have an annual budget, and a longer term planning horizon for major expenditures, say three years. It is impossible to consider major investments, for example in computerization, unless a time scale longer than 12 months is taken into account. In addition, the practice manager is responsible for the day-to-day control of the expenditure, although not necessarily involved in the recording or authorization of specific expenditures and receipts.

In business organizations the budget has two functions. First, it acts as a financial tool, involving estimates of future expenditures, both capital and operating, and future income. This is obviously necessary to ensure that the business does not run into financial difficulties, and is the major means of providing guidance for individual managers. Secondly, as a planning tool, as a way of representing the priorities of the business.

The practice budget is, however, different from the budget of a business organization. In business organizations the budget is related to anticipated income from the scale of the firm's products or services. The practice's level of income is determined largely by the level of fees and allowances provided by the NHS, apart from any income from private patients. The 'price' is determined by the buyer, not the provider of the service. This makes it more difficult for the practice manager to predict future income, particularly over a period longer than 12 months. However, the preparation of a financial plan, including an annual budget, remains essential.

The first major resource required by the practice manager is money. The practice manager is also responsible for the provision of physical facilities:

support facilities, including reception facilities, and office facilities. These are the second resource available. The precise equipment required will vary from practice to practice, according to the size of the partnership, the length of the patient list, the frequency of patient visits to the surgery, the number and competence of staff, and other factors. The practice manager's concern is with 'fitness for purpose'. Consideration needs to be given to the costs of service and maintenance as well as to the costs of the initial purchase. Again, it is important to consider the overall requirements of the practice.

The third major resource is staff time, both the practice manager's own and that of other members of staff. The preparation of an annual and a weekly schedule is again the responsibility of the practice manager; time management is a significant management responsibility, frequently taught on management programmes. The preparation of an annual calendar should give the practice manager the opportunity to review the workings of the practice with the partners. The review should cover the work of the practice manager herself, as well as the work of other members of staff. The practice manager will also need a weekly timetable. The details of the weekly timetable may change throughout the year, but again should be agreed with the partner who acts as 'managing partner' for the practice.

The timetable of clinical staff, doctors, employed practice nurses and attached staff who may use practice premises at times (such as health visitors, district nurses, a speech therapist, clinical psychologist, etc.) dictate the work-load coming through. The need to plan support staff for these activities as well as the other office or administrative activities is referred to in the paragraphs below.

The weekly timetable should include provision for a regular partner meeting, to cover the workings of the practice. The meetings may be informal, but records should be kept by the practice manager to ensure that decisions are carried forward.

The allocation of resources should be closely tied to the priorities of the practice. However, it is important to remember that issues may be of considerable importance, even if they are never the top priority; office support facilities may never be the top of the list, but provide a necessary basis for the effectiveness of the overall practice. Resources need to be provided for the infrastructure in conventional financial or indeed in medical terms.

Securing compliance

Securing compliance refers to the process of ensuring that the practice manager's wishes are carried out by other staff. It is not enough to 'make decisions' or to say 'do this' and to assume that your wishes will be carried out. In large industrial organizations securing compliance is a major problem, involving complex systems of supervision. Securing compliance is easier in small organizations, like medical practices. The practice manager can use her own personality and knowledge of individuals to build up loyalty and willingness to co-operate amongst the staff – the practice manager is not a remote name. The practice manager should be able to treat the staff as individuals. However, compliance cannot be taken for granted even in small organizations; it has to be sought and kept actively. This may be more difficult in general practice than in other small organizations because of the wide variety of staff including many part-time staff, with very different backgrounds and interests – medical, nursing, secretarial, as well as cleaning and repair staff. The pressure of large numbers of patients in the surgery is a further source of tension, making it important for the practice manager to be sensitive to the individual needs of the staff. A common problem is that decisions made at practice meetings are not followed through so the practice manager has to secure 'compliance' amongst doctors with their own decisions. How is this achieved?

Staff work for different reasons, and respond to different approaches. The main reason for complying with the wishes of the practice manager is custom and practice: it is expected. However, practices can become inefficient if practice managers become careless and begin to take compliance for granted. Compliance can become only nominal and provide a poor basis for an effective practice. Staff who work in general practice may have different approaches to work from staff who work in other organizations, and therefore accept orders for different reasons. In particular, the image of a caring profession will be important to many members of staff, and the approach adopted by the practice manager should reflect that approach. This is important for administrative as well as for medical and nursing staff. Such administrative staff, secretaries, receptionists and clerks, may be especially important, particularly in London and the south of England, because here they could obtain jobs in quite different lines of work—perhaps less interesting, but also less stressful and more remunerative. Even whilst adopting a financially realistic approach, the practice manager should not forget this caring orientation.

Different staff supervisors have different styles, some more authoritarian than others. The supervisory style should reflect the personality of the practice manager, the orientations of the staff, and the particular working environment of general practice. The need to ensure calm working relationships when working under pressure means that a very authoritarian approach is likely to lead to major difficulties, and especially to high levels of staff turnover; it is very wasteful for the practice to lose staff, since it takes time to learn the particular ways of operating of different practices.

The details of staff management are discussed in Chapter 6. Here the concern is simply to stress the importance of paying attention to the need to ensure compliance, and to secure that compliance actively.

Monitoring performance

The practice manager needs to ensure that the practice is working both effectively and efficiently. Effectively means achieving the overall objectives of the practice, efficiently means achieving this at minimum cost. This involves monitoring the performance of the practice as a whole, and of individual members of staff. This can only be done if the objectives of the practice are clear, priorities established and roles and tasks clearly defined.

The establishment of the overall aims of the practice is the responsibility of the partners. The partners should also be responsible for agreeing the measures of performance established to monitor the overall performance of the practice. This is very similar to the audit of clinical activities that clinical staff are involved with. Just as they have to measure what they do to see if it can be done better so do administrative staff and very frequently the two activities are intertwined. The practice manager may suggest possible measures, or indicate why some possible measures are inappropriate, perhaps because it would be difficult to keep information in the form required. The practice manager should ensure that information is available to the partners in a form which enables them to see how the practice is doing, and in a form which they can readily understand. In monitoring performance, comparable figures from a previous year, or from a comparable practice if available, should be provided. Partners do not wish to be overburdened with information, but the provision of basic information quarterly, with the possibility of having it available monthly, is one possible approach.

The practice manager is responsible for monitoring the performance of individual members of staff. She should avoid too heavy an emphasis upon formal monitoring of performance, because staff then begin to work to the performance criteria rather than to the requirements of the job, ignoring important parts of the job which may happen not to be measured. Formal monitoring should also be less necessary in a small organization than in a large organization, because the manager in a small organization has the possibility of directly observing the work of individual members of staff. However, increasing government concern with the costs of general practice may lead to the establishment of formal criteria of assessment for staff, as a condition for the reimbursement of costs, even if the assessment is unnecessary in terms of the practical operation of the practice. In the long run formal schemes of job evaluation may be established, which would involve assessments of the levels of skill and experience required, as well as the actual difficulty of the job. In the short run, practice managers should discuss systematically the performance of individual members of staff with the staff concerned at least once a year. This discussion should review the individuals's work thoughout the year, and should be separate from any discussion of salary, promotion or regrading.

The practice is a business, as well as a public service. The performance of the practice as a business will therefore have to be monitored. Such monitoring should focus on the performance of the practice against the budget. Comparisons of performance against budget may be made monthly or quarterly in business organizations; a similar frequency might be appropriate for a large practice.

Watching the outside world

The individual practice is a small part of a large organization. Its fortunes are very directly dependent upon its links with the outside world; hospitals, NHS administrative agencies, public health authorities, local authorities, other medical practitioners, as well as patients; the full range of relevant institutions is touched upon in later chapters. The doctors have a wide range of links with the medical world but it is also the practice manager's job to maintain contacts with the outside world, especially the non-medical world, and to be informed about changes which affect the practice. She must know what changes are being made by the DHA, for example alterations of clinic times, changed access to diagnostic facilities, appointments of new consultants and published lists of waiting times. She must be aware of changes initiated by the FHSA and think how every alteration in the terms and conditions of service might influence practice activity now and in the longer term. She must also watch the journals that come in to the practice for many of these provide information about practice activity elsewhere. Finally, she must be aware of changes in the local community around the practice. There is a major danger that the practice manager will be too inward looking, at a time when major threats to the practice are likely to come from outside.

The practice manager must obviously be aware of changes in the NHS which are likely to affect the practice. Changes in the financial arrangements governing the practice will have a direct impact upon the job of the practice manager. Closer monitoring of the financial performance will have a direct impact upon the practice manager, requiring the provision of more financial information than has been required in the past. Full budgetary responsibility for the individual practice would involve a very substantial increase in the responsibilities of the practice manager. Changes in the NHS will require the attention of the partners in the practice; but it will be the responsibility of the practice manager to ensure that up-to-date, accurate and full information is available to the partnership.

Other changes in the outside world will have a major impact upon the practice. Some of the changes will affect the 'patient mix' and therefore the likely pattern of surgery visits, for example if there is a major change in the age or social composition of the population in the area covered by the practice. New housing developments, or even simply changes in the price of houses in the district, may have significant implications for the practice. Many such changes will be known to the partners: but it is the practice manger's specific responsibility to be informed. Doctors are over-burdened with too much information.

To summarize, management is a process of decision making, involving seven elements.

1   Establishing objectives.
2   Defining roles, tasks and procedures.
3   Establishing priorities.
4   Securing and allocating resources.
5   Securing compliance.
6   Monitoring performance.
7   Watching the environment.

These basic management processes are the same, whether the manager is working in a large industrial organization or in a medical practice. Some of the elements require almost continuous awareness, especially monitoring performance and watching the environment. Some involve only occasional attention, establishing objectives and defining roles, tasks and procedures. However, each element requires attention at least annually.

Administration

Management is a decision-making activity, involving the choice between alternatives. Once decisions have been made, carrying them through involves administration. Administration is the establishment of rules and procedures, and applying those rules and procedures in particular cases. For example, specifying how repeat prescriptions should be dealt with, after the criteria have been laid down, and seeing that repeat prescriptions are made for individual patients in accordance with the rules specified.

Establishing rules and procedures and enforcing them may be bureaucratic, and bureaucracy is unpopular, especially with patients. Practice managers are therefore faced with the problem of balancing the requirements of administrative efficiency against the pressure to treat patients as individual, special cases. Too little flexibility is inhumane, too much flexibility leads to favouritism and difficulties in overall patient handling. It is necessary to judge when a patient's claim for priority attention is justified or not. Different practices will have different procedures and ways of administering the procedures, influenced by the partners and, especially, by the practice manager. Experience in non-medical organizations suggests five general comments.

Firstly, rules and procedures can only be developed when things happen regularly; it is impossible to develop rules for the unexpected, and a waste of time to develop rules for things which happen very infrequently. When establishing procedures it is necessary to consider how predictable an event is, and how often it occurs. The medical support, office and reception area activities of general practice involve large numbers of predictable and frequent events, and it is therefore desirable, and economical in time, to develop clear and relatively extensive formal procedures.

Secondly, the impact on staff of methods of administration needs to be considered. The development of rigid rules and procedures limits the scope for the exercise of initiative and discretion by practice staff. If they are always required to do exactly what the rule book tells them to do they are less likely to be willing, or able, to assume direct responsibility, even in an emergency, than if they are encouraged to make their own decisions.

However, practice staff are dealing with patients under stress, and it may be helpful to staff to have the rule book to rely upon when under pressure from patients, to 'know where they stand'. It is much easier, and more acceptable to say that 'the rules don't allow it' than to say 'I don't allow it'. Examples will include the rules about making appointments, responding to requests for home visits, patients speaking to doctors on the telephone, handling emergencies and so on. Moreover, there is a major need for continuity when large numbers of part-time staff are employed; this requires carefully worked out and clear procedures which can be relatively quickly learned. The chances of mistakes occurring through lack of knowledge of the practice are high, especially when large numbers of part-time staff are employed together.

Thirdly, the impact of administration on patients needs to be considered. Patients have conflicting wishes; the wish to be treated as special, as an individual, and the wish to be treated the same as everybody else, fairly. The first wish requires leaving a wide range of discretion to individual members of staff (for example on how urgently to make an appointment). The second wish involves specifying the rules fully (for example saying that priority appointments may only be made under specified circumstances).

Discretion must be given to staff to deal with emergencies, and to decide when an emergency is a real emergency. On the other hand, it is easier for a patient to complain that he or she was discriminated against and treated unfairly when there are no rules which state how a patient should be treated; the rules provide the criteria for judging whether the patient was treated fairly or not.

Fourthly, the impact of methods of administration upon the practice itself, and especially the ability to assess how efficiently the practice is working, needs to be considered. If procedures are unclear it is difficult to know whether 'best practice' is being followed or not, and if staff time is being used efficiently. This links in with the importance of monitoring performance.

Finally, formal procedures will be increasingly important as the NHS concerns itself more with 'good management' and 'value for money'. Practices will need to demonstrate to outsiders that they are providing value for money. It is easier to demonstrate 'value for money' if there are clear administrative procedures than if wide areas are left to individual discretion. Practices which leave large areas of discretion to individual members of staff, and fail to provide adequate training, will be especially likely to be criticized. It is also the best protection against charges from outside that mistakes have been made and care not provided of an adequate standard.

The development of information technology is having a direct impact upon practice administration. Repeat prescribing is now computerized in nearly 50% of all practices. Some form of clinical record-keeping is computerized in 30% and systems for managing appointment systems and financial systems are being introduced. These do not often make less work and they usually make more, but they do improve the quality of what is done and make it possible to obtain data about what is going on within the practice for audit purposes. Newer and more sophisticated systems will be required as the role of general practice continues to expand and as links are developed between data held by DHAs, FHSAs and the practice itself. Information on performance will be required both for good practice and in order to demonstrate good practice.

Conclusion

The general practice is a small organization, working within the framework of a very large organization. This is the type of pattern which many large business organizations are trying to establish as the most efficient form of organization 'small within large'. This presents the practice manager with many opportunities, as well as difficulties. This concluding section outlines the opportunities and difficulties which face the practice manager compared with the manager in a large industrial organization.

The practice manager is a member of a small team. She is able to know the other members of the team as individuals, and to build up close working relations with them. This makes it easier to develop commitment to the practice. With a small team it is possible to develop a flexible approach to work, with members of the practice encouraged to learn about the whole range of practice activities. Small size means that there is no need to waste time passing information up a chain of command, and waiting perhaps for months for decisions. Personal relationships, and personal feelings, are important. At the same time, the practice has access to the resources of a very large organization, the NHS. This is a source of expertise, advice and assistance, as well as finance.

Although the practice is small, it is not simple. Although there are only a small number of staff, they have very different skills, and they are not interchangeable. There are therefore limits to the job flexibility which is possible. Moreover, the pressures under which doctors work mean that it is not always possible to secure their attention for practice management problems, and to obtain necessary decisions. Finally, the NHS imposes many requirements upon practices, not all of which are helpful to the practice itself, as well as providing resources.

The practice manager is a 'negotiator' between the different groups involved in the practice – the partners, the staff, the patients, the NHS. Each has to be satisfied if the practice is to work effectively. The partners are the major 'stakeholders' and if they are not satisfied the practice manager is not likely to remain in the practice for very long. But the other stakeholders need to be satisfied also in the long run if the practice is to survive. The practice manager therefore needs to consider the interests of all stakeholders and to consider how to reconcile their often conflicting interests.

This task of negotiation is similar to that of managers in other organizations. However, there are five features which make the task of the practice manager different from the task of other managers.

Firstly, she is responsible for a wide range of tasks, which would be divided between different departments in a larger organization – finance, personnel, purchasing, office management, relations with the public. This makes the job in some ways easier, since she does not have to consult with a wide range of other managers. But it also makes it more demanding, since she is responsible for such a variety of relationships.

Secondly, she is responsible for a wide range of staff – nursing, secretarial, cleaning and maintenance. This again requires awareness of a wide range of issues; different grades of staff have different skills, interests, and pay scales. If large numbers of part-time staff are employed there is the additional problem of arranging work schedules. Staff management is especially important because of the importance of staff sensitivity to patient needs.

Thirdly, she will be involved in dealing with the general public, at a time when they are experiencing personal stress. This is likely to lead to tension in the reception area, especially if the doctors are unable to keep to the appointments timetable. The practice manger will be working 'in public', and may be called upon to handle tensions between her staff and members of the public.

Fourthly, the practice manager has little control over the major factors which determine the income of the practice. The business manager is able to determine the price of his product according to the costs of the production, the prices charged by competitors, and generally by 'what the market will bear'. The practice manager is tied to a scale of fees and reimbursements determined by the FHSA, and in commercial terms is operating with one hand tied behind her back. She is able to influence the expenditures of the practice, but not to have an equivalent influence on the income.

Finally, the practice manager has little influence over the institutional context in which the practice operates. The context is provided by the NHS, and the NHS operates within a complex legislative framework. The practice manager has to be aware of the ways in which the NHS affects the practice, but has little opportunity to influence the wider organization. There is little opportunity for the practice manager to look for new markets!

The practice manager is, then a special kind of manager. She is required to perform the same management tasks as other managers but she is operating in a unique environment, with its own constraints and opportunities. The remainder of this book provides advice on how to manage in these special circumstances.

3 The Role of the Practice Manager

IT is extremely difficult to give a universal description of a practice manager's role because the title means something different to each practice. At one end of the scale there are those who have been promoted through the ranks and perform a senior administrative role; at the other end of the scale are those who perform a wider management role with considerable responsibilities. This chapter concentrates on the practice manager who is given sufficient scope by the partners to manage all aspects of the practice, and who is expected to participate in all practice activities. This does not mean that the practice manager acts in isolation when making and effecting decisions. However, it does mean that the practice manager uses personal and technical skills to assume the role of management adviser to the partners in the decision-making process.

The practice manager is neither partner nor the usual employee. Herein lie both strength and frustration. The strength comes from the ability to act as mediator between the partners and the practice staff, communicating views and decisions both upwards and downwards. The frustration often arises from not having another person within the practice who understands the unique position of the practice manager and who can identify with the concerns that the manager may have about the direction in which the practice is moving. The practice manager listens to everyone else's problems and is expected to provide solutions but who listens to hers?

Box 3.1 is a sample job description of a practice manager, including a brief discussion of each heading.

Objective statement

The initial statement outlines what the practice manager should be trying to achieve, and will vary according to the wishes of the partners. Each section of the job description should relate back to this aim to ensure a cohesive role for the practice manager to fulfil.

Box 3.1: Sample job description for practice manager

Job description

The practice manager shall be responsible for the efficient, effective and safe administrative and financial management of the practice, and ensure the well-being of patients, doctors and staff, and the successful smooth running of the practice.

Partnership secretary

- compile the agenda for partnership meetings
- convene, attend, participate in and be responsible for the minutes of each meeting
- organize and participate in all staff meetings
- arrange all financial controls and reports
- arrange confidential partnerships matters (eg mortgages, agreements, partners' salaries, partnership contracts and retainers)
- arrange all administration regarding the Family Health Services Authority (FHSA)
- act as management adviser to the partners

The partners

- compile and publish the night and weekend duty rota
- instruct trainees and medical students in practice management
- personally support the partners in matters relating to management
- be responsible for adequate medical cover and arrange locums when necessary
- remind partners of agreed practice policy
- arrange regular audit, diary and clinical meetings, including the invitation of appropriate consultants or health professionals
- act as personnel manager to the partners

The staff

- ensure proper conditions of employment, to include current employment legislation and recognized good practice
- recruit and maintain an efficient and cost-effective level of staffing
- instigate and arrange a staff training programme
- be responsible for an effective appraisal system and any resulting training or disciplinary procedures
- maintain adequate relief staff to cover holidays or absence
- communicate agreed practice policy to staff and introduce systems to support such policies

Box 3.1: *continued*

- ensure that all staff are aware of the importance of protecting any confidential information about patients, doctors or colleagues

The patients

- meet all prospective patients and discuss their allocation to a doctor
- welcome new patients to the practice and give them health questionnaires and appointments for new patient health checks
- deal with patient complaints
- deal with internal transfers of doctor
- be involved with the Patient Participation Group, either as a point of contact or as an organizer
- maintain informative and up-to-date notice boards

General administration

- ensure compliance with all statutory and legal regulations
- effect and maintain insurance policies: public and third party liability, employers' liability, premises and equipment
- ensure security of personnel and property
- be responsible for supplies, both medical and administrative
- manage buildings, extensions, repairs, decorations, fixtures and fittings, gardening and maintenance of exterior
- maintain high standards of hygiene
- arrange systems management of the computer; all aspects of training, development, applications and integration

Finance and accounts

- liaise with practice accountant to produce annual audited accounts
- prepare and present financial plans for approval
- supervise and monitor practice ledgers, petty cash, bank reconciliations, cash flow forecasts, and income and expenditure plans
- advise on and administer the drawings of the partners and appropriate salary scales for staff
- supervise all Pay-As-You-Earn (PAYE) and National Insurance (NI) contributions
- submit accounts for all non-GMS work
- produce a detailed quarterly breakdown of income and expenditure

---

Box 3.1: *continued*

Entertaining and social

- arrange any social function that may be held to mark a special practice occasion
- organize any public relations exercises with outside agencies or visitors to the practice
- attend any local function as deemed necessary by the practice, during normal working hours

Confidential matters

- deal personally with any confidential matter about the practice or the partners and reports to any official or professional body.
- perform any duty specifically designated by the partners as being properly the responsibility of the practice manager

---

Partnership secretary

This is perhaps the traditional function of the practice manager. The 1990s have brought about great changes within general practice, and the role of the 'minute taker' at practice meetings is being replaced by the need for management support and advice. Most practices have accepted that the partners are too busy providing a full range of medical services to patients to be able to become involved in the nuts and bolts of running a practice. This has given practice managers an opportunity to extend their role and assume responsibilities that were once the exclusive domain of the partners, and has helped to make the practice manager's job more interesting and rewarding.

The partners

Keeping a group of doctors in line is probably the hardest part of the job! The most sensitive area of contact with the partners is when they need to be reminded of practice policy; in other words, when they do something that is clearly out of line with current agreements. This takes every ounce of a practice manager's skill of tact and diplomacy. It is essential that personal feelings are set aside to ensure parity of treatment; for example, you might be tempted to let a favourite partner take time off when you would not consider letting your least favourite do the same. Credibility relies upon parity of enforcement of policies. Doctors are trained to care for others, but they are notoriously bad at looking after themselves or giving their families priority occasionally. Here the practice manager has a vital role to play in maintaining an eye on the partners as people as well as doctors.

The staff

The practice manager's responsibilities to the staff are clear. They must have contracts, training, appraisals and be taught to work well as a team as well as recognizing their individual strengths. There is no doubt that a happy working atmosphere will reduce absences and enhance staff pride in their work and loyalty to the practice.

The patients

We should never forget that the patients are the reason for the practice being in existence. It is too easy to let the administration and government imposi-tions get in the way of keeping in touch with our patients' needs and wishes. The practice manager should seize any opportunity to meet and talk with patients to keep abreast of the practice's public image and to respond to their demands.

General administration

This area is very straightforward, but time consuming. A great deal of this administration can be effectively delegated to other members of the practice team. For example, there is no reason why the practice nurses should not assume responsibility for the treatment room supplies and be taught to work to an agreed budget. The same applies to office stationery and domestic consumables. A good diary system will make sure that insurance policy renewals are not overlooked.

The greatest impact on practice administration has been the introduction of computers, and the practice manager needs to control and monitor the implications for each and every practice system.

Finance and accounts

When it comes to financial matters, the practice manager has help close at hand in the shape of the accountant and the bank manager. Both are specially trained to understand general business finance, and an attachment to either, or both, is time well spent to obtain an overall picture. The same applies to the finance officers at the FHSA. We are encouraged to produce cash flow forecasts and to monitor income and expenditure on a regular basis. Without such information we cannot channel our efforts appropriately and may waste time looking into problems that do not even exist.

Entertaining and social

The practice manager is usually the person who decides the frequency of social events, and the format that they should take. It could be anything from a 'get together' at someone's house to a formal annual dinner. There are also practice occasions that need to be celebrated; for example, a partner retiring. These functions can be a positive team-building exercise if handled correctly. It is an opportunity for the practice manager to show some flair and imagination.

Confidential matters

There are any number of things that do not fit readily into any particular category. The practice manager's discretion is often needed to deal with a situation quickly and effectively.

Resource management

The essence of management is the proper deployment of available resources. It does not matter if these resources are physical, financial or personnel, the principles are the same. No task can be undertaken until a complete breakdown and costing has been done. If the benefits outweigh the costs, it is 'cost-effective'.

Box 3.2:   A cost-effectiveness calculation

To produce an in-house practice brochure:

Computer	£2000
Software package	£500
40 staff hours @ £5.50	£220
Paper for 1000 brochures	£200
Total	£2920

Professional quote for 1000 brochures	£1000

It is estimated that 1000 brochures would be one year's supply.

The decision to be made is whether the capital investment in new equipment is worth it, if a printing company could be used for three years before the benefit is gained.

Box 3.3:   A cost-benefit calculation

The 1992 Health and Safety (Display Screen Equipment) Regulations demand that any new workstation from 1 January 93 must conform to certain standards. A new computer terminal was delivered in April 1993 and must comply with the legislation, which will mean a new adjustable operator's chair costing £200.

The benefit is prevention because it concerns the health of the member of staff using the new terminal, but there is no option.

However, there may be times when the costs are justified because there is no other option available, or because it is a legal requirement.

The practice manager must ensure that value for money is being gained from every single asset that the practice may possess, and this includes protecting investment in the building or equipment by insurance or regular maintenance.

The largest single investment of any practice is the building, and it should be fully utilized to ensure that income from items of service is maximized. The rooms themselves need to be well planned to prevent any time being wasted in finding or using equipment. If there are parts of the day when surgeries or treatment rooms are empty, could they be used for additional health promotion clinics? Could they be rented out to other health professionals on a sessional basis?

The second largest investment is in practice staff. The cash limit imposed by the FHSA on funding for practice staff is likely to get tighter, so each practice needs to plan ahead and use every opportunity to review, and possibly re-structure, its staffing levels. When someone leaves or retires, it is not enough simply to replace them. Use the vacancy to review each person's responsibilities and look at existing staff to undertake the core jobs that need to be done before automatically recruiting another person. In most practices there is some slack that can be used; that is, quiet times when additional administration can be done by current staff. Similarly, there are often duplications that can be eliminated. This is a very complex issue as each member of staff needs to be treated as an individual and helped to reach his or her full potential. The practice manager should not staff the practice based on historical demands, but look to the future and anticipate the changing demands. This is dealt with more fully in Chapter 4.

Suggestions to eliminate waste and make savings often come from the people actually doing the job. By making information about certain items of expenditure (eg stationery) available to the administrative staff they will be able to suggest ways of cutting down the bills. This can be taken a step further by allocating a budget and making one person responsible for ordering routine items. This kind of involvement achieves two aims: first, it delegates one job from the practice manager's desk, and secondly it makes staff more responsible for their actions. The result can only be a positive one.

Leadership skills

Effective leadership is not just about giving orders and leading from the front, only to find out that the troops are not behind you!

The strongest leadership is often not perceived as such because it goes on quietly and efficiently all the time. It is a combination of example, knowing the staff and partners well enough to have their honest opinions, personal credibility, mutual trust, patience and research. A practice manager who rushes in to come up with a solution without discussion with all parties usually comes to grief and ends up losing face. Not an ideal way to improve credibility.

There are three fundamental issues that an effective leader considers before making a decision or taking any action: to achieve the objective; to develop the individual; and to strengthen the team.

1   The ability to achieve any given objective is important to the efficiency of the business. However, there are other positive benefits to the morale of the team and a sense of pride in a job well done.
2   The needs of every individual must be recognized if they are to be motivated and encouraged to develop their potential. The status acquired by association with the successful conclusion of a given project will ensure their co-operation in the future.
3   The cohesive team will always achieve more than any individual and produce a particular kind of group dynamics. The team that works well is mutually supporting and well motivated.

These issues are interdependent and the practice manager must consider all three elements when considering any task. To ignore one will have an adverse effect on the others. The model shown in Figure 3.1 represents the ideal leadership style.

Co-ordinator and facilitator

The practice manager is the contact point for all the groups of personnel essential to the well-being of the patients (Figure 3.2). Many of them have limited opportunities or the time available for direct contact. In this respect

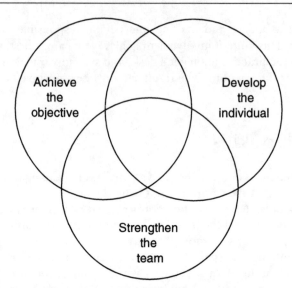

Figure 3.1:   A model of the ideal leadership style.

the practice manager has incredible power, and must report facts and situations in an accurate and unbiased way, offering personal opinions only when asked.

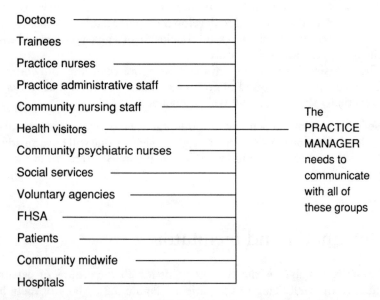

Figure 3.2:   The practice manager needs to communicate with all these groups.

The practice manager is also the person within the practice who has the authority to make things happen; that is, to make staff, time and resources available. It is quite usual for the practice manager to have a specified limit to expenditure before obtaining the consent or approval of the partners. This, combined with regular contact with all parties, puts the practice manager firmly into the facilitator role.

It would be all too easy to take on all the practice problems and innovations personally, but time will not permit. Here the practice manager must learn to delegate effectively, often by handing back a situation to the person who raised it with a clear plan of how to set about finding a solution.

Delegation is not simply about giving clear directions. It needs to include a degree of monitoring, encouragement and support. Whilst all this takes precious time, it does set the scene for the future and over a period of time the staff will come to think for themselves and start raising possible solutions along with their problems. The danger is in being seen to be uninterested; staff may find another person within the practice in whom to confide their concerns or take their suggestions. This is obviously undesirable as it will undermine the practice manager's personal credibility and authority if it becomes the norm.

The example given in Box 3.4 is of a simple practice system that is going wrong. However, it demonstrates the amount of delegation that can be employed without losing touch or showing lack of interest in a routine problem.

Routine problems with mundane tasks must be given due importance because these tend to cause the greatest disruption to practice life. There is little more annoying than finding that a vital supply has run out and no one seems to be responsible for checking or re-ordering. When these problems arise, they need to be dealt with quickly and in such a way that they are unlikely to arise again. In this way we slowly improve the overall efficiency of the practice and release time to spend on more major issues.

Poor communication is the biggest single inhibitor to efficiency and the practice manager should ensure that each group is given opportunities to meet regularly. This includes checking that appropriate people are available, a suitable venue is free, an agenda is prepared and circulated, refreshments (depending on the time of day) are organized, someone is nominated to take notes, a chairperson nominated in advance and minutes are circulated after the meeting. The practice manager does not need to attend every meeting simply for the sake of it, but will evaluate the potential contribution and subject matter before making a decision. Often it is enough to create the opening for dialogue and monitor any subsequent decisions.

Box 3.4:   Delegation helps problem solving

Situation:

The administrative staff are complaining that the laboratory forms are constantly running out, and the hospital never send the amount requested.

Possible solution:

Is there a real problem?
Establish the quantity of forms needed on a
weekly basis by carrying out a survey.
(Administrative staff)

↓

Discuss results of survey
(Practice manager and administrative staff)

↓

Write to the hospital manager, outlining the
problem and enclosing survey results. Request a
weekly standing order of forms.
(Practice manager)

↓

Monitor all deliveries of forms.
(Administrative staff)

↓

Give feedback on any problems with the system.
*(Administrative staff to practice manager; practice
manager to hospital manager)*

↓

Advise of outcome.
(Practice manager to administrative staff)

Conclusion:

The practice manager has given due attention to the problem: delegated the research and monitoring to the staff who raised the issue and encouraged them to take some responsibility in finding a satisfactory solution. The staff also have the opportunity to raise the issue again.

Management style

Each practice manager has a unique personality and should use this to evolve a management style. The emphasis should be on outcome, the means being left to each practice manager – although there are recommended routes. There are many courses and seminars on management run by a variety of bodies, all of whom have powerful messages to deliver. However, trying to adopt a style that is uncomfortable will quickly be perceived as insincere by colleagues, partners and staff. The successful manager uses several styles depending upon the situation; this is a strength, as it demonstrates the ability to review each issue on merit. There will be a preferred approach and it is this that gives a practice manager a reputation of consistency, and the staff and partners will come to rely upon a particular response, especially when dealing with a sensitive problem.

The wimp

The 'wimp' is best typified by the phrase 'anything for a quite life'. This style, if carried to an extreme, will mean that the manager gets submerged by more forceful personalities within the practice. Difficult issues will probably never be faced because the trauma involved in managing change will be felt to be too distressing.

The egotist

The egotist will constantly seek attention and approval from the partners. Good ideas from others will be relayed to superiors as though they are the manager's own. The danger is a concentration on tasks that will be noticed at the expense of the basic, and hidden, things that contribute to an efficient unit. There will be isolation from subordinates and the reputation of being a 'creep'.

The headless chicken

This describes the 'reactive manager'; that is, someone who spends the majority of the day dealing with a crisis. The danger is the feeling of having lost control of one's own actions because all energies are concentrated on sorting out the problems of others. This is perhaps the easiest to change by learning to set aside time to plan and to learn to delegate effectively.

The sheep

This type of manager is comfortable following the orders of the partners, and often does not make personal views known because of either a lack of confidence or disinterest. This complete lack of personal input into decisions could result in the practice deciding that the role is not needed! Staff are unlikely to use the manager as anything other than a route to have their views heard by the partners.

The bully

The bully simply bulldozes through all obstacles and objections. Whilst it may be effective in achieving objectives, it will do little to build any kind of team spirit. There are occasions when this is the only course of action, but it is best limited to legal and contractual impositions by outside agencies.

The friend

This type of manager does not really want to manage but would prefer to be 'one of the girls'. Decisions that are likely to prove unpopular will be avoided at all costs, and the acceptance of responsibility will be low. This manager's strength will be in personnel matters when a caring and understanding response is called for. The danger is in the possibility of being manipulated by the staff.

The thinker

The usual reply will be 'I'll think about that' but resulting action is unlikely. This manager will have plans, usually written, for everything in the future but will have achieved very little in practical terms. Staff will eventually bypass the manager if a problem needs urgent, and visible, action.

The consultant

This is probably the ideal style to adopt. It combines seeking the opinions and advice of others before recommending a particular course of action. Such decisions are unlikely to be overturned because the team feel that they have contributed. This type of manager will build a cohesive team and command respect from all parties.

Experience and a detailed knowledge of each member of the team will help the practice manager to adopt an appropriate style for each situation. This understanding will facilitate the review of all information before making a decision, and turn each major decision into a team-building opportunity. It is essential for the practice manager to take advantage of the 'neither partner, nor staff' status to be seen to be fair and capable of making unbiased judgements.

Business planning

We tend to forget that general practice is a business, and even the smallest practice has a considerable turnover. A 'business plan' is the term used for the document that outlines the future aims and direction of the practice. In industry and commerce this would equate to the annual stocktake. Although the sound is daunting, much of the information needed is readily at hand in a well-organized unit. Like all large tasks, it can be broken down into component parts, and information collected under each heading.

Workload
- list size
- consultation and visiting rates
- referral rates
- clinical audit.

Personnel
- number of partners
- regular locums
- staffing numbers and categories
- attached staff.

Premises
- is there sufficient space?
- utilization of space
- owned or rented?

Equipment
- medical
- office
- domestic.

Finance
- comparison with intended remuneration for partners
- comparison with average item of service income figures
- analysis of expenditure.

The majority of this information will already have been collected and published in the practice annual report. The information is factual and therefore provides a solid base from which to build a business plan.

The next step is to set aside a series of practice meetings to devote exclusively to formulating the business plan. The concept of 'away days' is currently in vogue and has merit. The key personnel within the practice need to sit and discuss every issue in detail and reach some kind of agreement if the plan is to be adhered to in the future. This is done most effectively away from the interruptions of the surgery, and preferably in pleasant surroundings to encourage all parties to feel relaxed and open with one another.

The business plan will remain just a document unless it is acceptable to all as the way forward. The discussion of sensitive issues is inevitable, and a skilled facilitator will defuse conflict and turn it into constructive criticism.

It is essential that the business plan, once formulated, becomes a dynamic document that is regularly reviewed and updated in line with progress and developments. It can be an invaluable tool, and a steadying influence if the practice starts moving in a different direction. Ideally, it should be placed as an item on the practice meeting agenda every three or six months.

A tried and tested management technique is to devise a SWOT analysis. This stands for Strengths, Weaknesses, Opportunities and Threats, and is usually used in the format shown in Figure 3.3. It combines the factual information with other factors that may influence the practice, and provides

Strengths	Weaknesses
Opportunities	Threats

Figure 3.3:   An outline for a SWOT analysis.

Strengths	Weaknesses
- high standard of care - good local reputation - well-motivated staff - low patient turnover - 'preferred doctor' seen - strong management - evening and Saturday surgeries offered - training practice - regular audit meetings - good communications - adjacent to Community Hospital - attached Community Staff on site	- no nurse-run clinics - cramped administrative area - inadequate staff training - low item of service income - partners' lack of interest in practice management - few outside commitments - demanding patients - all male partners
Opportunities	**Threats**

- new housing estate planned in practice
  area
- local businesses opening that may
  need a medical officer
- land adjacent to practice for sale
- full-time senior partner retiring
- FHSA offering some funds for staff
  training
	- new single-handed doctor has applied
	  to start a practice in new estate
	- car park needs resurfacing

Figure 3.4:   An example of a completed SWOT analysis.

an opportunity to highlight any openings for the practice to develop its full potential. A completed SWOT analysis could look like Figure 3.4.

Once the analysis is complete an action plan can be prepared to deal with each point. The skill is to preserve and develop the strengths, correct the weaknesses, minimize and prepare for threats, and take advantage of opportunities. In other words, the SWOT analysis should be dealt with as a whole entity and the practice manager will normally be the one to monitor progress.

The action of preparing a written document will focus the attention, and there may be some obvious links. For example:

- The practice has all male partners, which is seen as a weakness. When the senior partner retires, there will be an opportunity to replace him with one or two female doctors.
- The FHSA funding for staff training will eliminate another perceived weakness of inadequate staff training.

The SWOT analysis and business planning are 75% research and preparation. To gather the senior members of the practice team together for a day, half-day or a series of evening meetings is expensive; this is wasted if a decision cannot be made because background information is needed. Apart from the monetary implications, the impetus and enthusiasm to get a plan formulated and agreed will also be lost. Therefore, successful planning will depend on the practice manager's ability to anticipate the questions and have the answers ready.

The business plan becomes dynamic when it is translated into a series of objectives and action plans.

Setting objectives

There is no doubt that the most successful companies, multinational or small, have a strong corporate image. This does not happen by accident, but by strong leadership and shared aims with all employees. The practice manager's role is to create practical plans to achieve the objectives, and then follow them through.

The reasons for setting objectives are:

- to improve and maintain performance
- to establish a common aim to unite the partners
- to provide a training tool for staff
- to set aims that can be communicated to attached community staff and outside agencies.
- to set aims for the practice team to be proud of
- for team-building
- to generate a feeling of 'ownership' by all members of the practice
- to publish the objectives in practice brochures
- to develop individuals by using their skills to achieve the objectives
- to provide an opportunity to give praise when objectives have been achieved
- to give clear guidelines for members of the team to use to self-regulate their actions
- to maintain discipline
- to encourage all members of the team to contribute to the overall success and progress of the practice.

Setting objectives can be a totally positive exercise, with no disadvantages.

To explain the process of setting objectives we will refer to the completed SWOT analysis and take the 'weaknesses' section as an example.

Weaknesses

No nurse-run clinics

Objective: to train practice nurses to enable them to run their own clinics to monitor diabetic patients routinely.

Plan:

- evaluate suitable diabetic care courses for nurses
- book for at least one nurse to attend the most appropriate course
- identify the number of diabetic patients registered with the practice
- devise a protocol that is agreed by all doctors and nurses
- set up an effective call and re-call system for diabetic patients
- audit the care of diabetic patients
- review protocols, if necessary
- train all practice nurses to give cover for absence and increase flexibility.

Cramped administrative area

Objective: to improve the use of space in the administrative area.

Plan:

- brain-storm the problem with all staff working in the area
- invite an office design consultant to advise on possible alterations
- review office equipment and identify any future changes (word processing on existing computer terminals will make typewriters redundant)
- evaluate costs and benefits of all suggestions before making changes.

Inadequate staff training

Objective: to identify training needs and introduce regular staff training sessions.

Plan:

- agree desirable standard of staff skills with partners and staff
- use job descriptions as a means of identifying training needs
- discuss areas of concern with each member of staff, preferably during an appraisal interview
- devise outside courses for experience staff
- plan a suitable time and day to hold training sessions
- divide staff into small groups with similar needs
- use experienced staff to train the inexperienced
- plan the training programme in advance
- maintain enthusiasm by including some 'nice to know' topics as well as the 'need to know' ones
- use job swopping and attachments, where appropriate
- include all members of the team as trainers
- evaluate effectiveness at the next appraisal
- hold an open forum after six months to hear the staff views on the training to date

- keep detailed records of training to cost the exercise and possibly to claim reimbursement from the FHSA.

It should be clear from these examples that even the most straightforward objective requires a great deal of management input and teamwork to translate it into action. All objectives need to be written down and available to the team; by doing this they are unlikely to get filed away and forgotten. It is also possible to delegate certain objectives to members of the team, especially if one person's enthusiasm can be harnessed to encourage others.

It might be worth putting a poster, giving all the practice objectives, in a prominent place to keep them firmly in everyone's mind!

4 The Personnel Management of the Team

'PERSONNEL management' is the term used to describe the way we deal with staff during their employment, and sometimes after they have left. It encompasses every member of the team, including the partners and the attached community staff. The best indicator of good personnel management is a positive 'atmosphere', impossible to quantify but immediately obvious if it is lacking.

The negative signs will be apparent first because they surface in the form of conflict, and they need to be dealt with quickly before they become too deep-rooted for the trend to be reversed. Dissatisfaction tends to feed upon itself and there are always one or two individuals willing to keep feelings running high in the rest of the team.

Symptoms of poor personnel management

- Lateness
- No acceptance of responsibility
- Petty bickering
- Grumbles about others
- 'What's in it for me' attitude
- Lack of interest in patients and colleagues
- No participation in meetings
- Unhelpful, even obstructive, to others
- Rudeness
- Uncommunicativeness
- Small problems get out of hand
- The formation of cliques

Good personnel management is a combination of common sense and trustworthy systems. Although even the best systems work well only if they are adhered to religiously, just having one is not enough. This chapter is intended as a guide through the employment cycle, starting with recruitment and ending with leaving procedures.

Recruitment

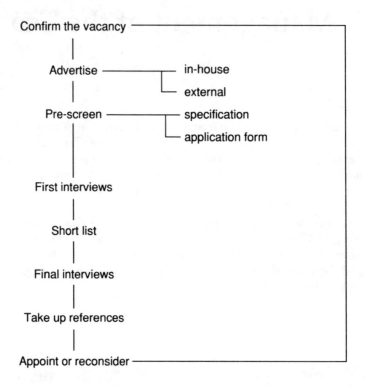

Figure 4.1:   Steps to filling a vacancy.

Confirm the vacancy

It is frequently the most basic things that get forgotten in any complicated process. It does not matter if it is a new post or a vacancy as a result of labour turnover, it is essential that the vacancy is reviewed before any recruitment begins. There must be agreement about the required hours, job title, purpose and responsibilities. It needs to be established if the vacancy is going to be on a short-term or long-term contract.

It is too easy to replace staff with someone else working exactly the same hours and performing the same duties, instead of seeing the vacancy as an opportunity to prepare for future demands.

Most FHSAs are allocating staff budgets to practices, which eliminates the obligation to seek permission before altering the staffing or advertising a new post. The staffing budget represents 70% of gross salaries, 100% of the employers' National Insurance contributions and an agreed percentage 'uplift' to cover salary increases and increments. Each FHSA works in a slightly different way, so it is advisable to double-check what notification, if any, they require. The budget is a finite figure and if a practice overspends it must be prepared to pay the excess from practice funds.

When the details of the vacancy are settled they should be written down in the form of a hand-out, circulated to staff and sent out with application forms later in the process.

In-house advertising

Making the full details of any anticipated recruitment available to the existing staff can often bring a few surprises, and solutions. Practices are predominantly staffed by women working part-time, and in the current economic climate more women need to work longer hours to supplement the family income. There may be part-time staff who wish to work full-time or job-share. To recruit from within has some attractions: ready-trained staff who are acceptable to the team and who will have a clear idea of the expectations and their own capability to do the proposed job. The only disadvantage is if an unsuitable member of staff applies, but regular appraisal discussions should leave everyone with a clear idea of their performance strengths and limitations. If this situation does arise, the only course of action is to tell the member of staff honestly, but kindly, why he or she will not be appointed.

External advertising

The normal places to advertise are the professional journals, and local and national newspapers. However, the FHSA might be willing to circulate notification of a vacancy, and the value of word of mouth should never be underestimated. Not only do the right quantity of applicants need to be attracted, but also they should have the right background and experience. Careful thought should be given to the most effective advertising medium. Costs will also have a bearing: as a general rule, the national newspapers are the most expensive, local papers are cheaper and some professional journals offer a free service. Maximum benefit needs to be gained from the advertisement because re-advertising will prove costly, in time as well as in money.

The first decision is whether to advertise 'lineage' or 'box'. The lineage is exactly as it sounds, and will appear in a column of similar advertisements. The box can be any number of lines deep and columns wide as is deemed necessary, and costs increase according to the size of the box. The box advert is usually more expensive than a lineage advert, but it can attract greater interest if it is made to be eye-catching.

DR SMITH AND PARTNERS
High Street Practice
Ambridge

have a permanent vacancy for a

PART-TIME MEDICAL SECRETARY

4 hours per day, Monday to Friday.
Saturdays on a rota of one per month.

This busy practice needs a competent and reliable person to assume responsibility for all communication to hospitals. Ability to work as part of a team essential. Salary will be based on previous experience.

Job description and application form available
from Mrs Brown, on 0222 334455.

Figure 4.2:   Sample newspaper advertisement.

The wording of the advertisement is extremely important because it must be seen to be open to all; that is, not discriminatory in any way for reasons of sex, colour, race or religion. It must also attract at least one suitable candidate, and discourage those who cannot fulfil certain aspects of the job, such as the hours. Some criteria will be negotiable, others essential. This should be communicated via the advertisement.

The aim is to achieve a balance of information in the advertisement that will encourage a number of applicants, not to narrow the field by being too specific. All newspapers offer the facility of a box number, which some practices may prefer to use. The main purpose in doing so would be to conceal the name of the practice that requires new staff, perhaps because of internal politics or because the address of the practice may be off-putting.

The advertisement shown in Figure 4.2 is intended to convey:

- town centre
- permanent vacancy
- 4 hours per day, which are negotiable
- some unsocial hours, ie Saturdays
- clearly defined task
- the applicant will be fully occupied during the 20 hours
- strong secretarial skills needed
- a key post that demands personal commitment
- team skills required, eg good communication, flexibility

- newly qualified or experienced medical secretaries will be considered
- an untrained person would not be considered
- salary negotiable.

Pre-screening

There must be some element of pre-screening, simply because no practice has sufficient time available to see every single applicant, especially as some will be unable to meet one or more of the basic criteria. Planning and information will help the applicants to self-eliminate, and save wasted interview time. The techniques available to assist this process are an agreed specification of the successful candidate and the application form.

Specification

A written specification should be prepared in advance of any interviews and used as part of the pre-screening. It can be for the exclusive use of the practice, or sent out to applicants with the application form. It can take the form of a check-list, or a slightly more personal letter that encompasses the main points.

The following points should be included, irrespective of the format:

- brief description of practice and working environment
- main areas of responsibility
- training, required and offered
- salary scale and review dates
- desired arrangement of hours
- level of fitness required
- personal qualities, eg
  - neat appearance
  - articulate
  - common sense
  - use initiative
  - open and friendly
- attainments, eg
  - legible handwriting
  - good telephone manner
  - relevant experience
- special skills, eg confidentiality
- physical circumstances, eg
  - live near practice
  - reliable transport.

'Core' application form

Post applied for:		
Surname:		
Forenames:		
Address:		
Postcode:	Tel. No:	
Date of birth:	Marital status:	
Are you currently employed? YES/NO		
If YES, complete the following: Name and address:		
Job title:		
Date started: Salary:		
Reasons for wishing to leave:		
Give details of previous employment during the past FIVE years:		
Name of employer:	From:	To:

Figure 4.3: Example of a 'core' application form.

How many days off work, through illness, have you taken in the last two years?	
Do you have any on-going health problems?	YES/NO
If YES, please describe:	

Please list any qualifications or examinations passed, with dates:	
Qualification:	Date:

continue on separate sheet, if necessary

Have you ever used a computer?	YES/NO
Can you use a word processor?	YES/NO
Are you willing to train to use a computer and/or word processor?	YES/NO

Please describe any experience you may have of working with the public, in a medical environment or in a position of responsibility:

Please give the names and addresses of two people who would be willing to provide a reference. They must have known you for a number of years and not be relatives:

Name:	Name:
Address:	Address:

Figure 4.3: *continued*

Application form

The application form (Figure 4.3) ensures that the practice keeps control and determines the information received by asking pertinent questions. It also allows like to be compared with like, without hidden bias. That is, elegant headed notepaper may be seen as an advantage over an application written on a page from a notebook. The application form is a levelling tool, although the standard of completion will have an influence on the assessor. To avoid having to design a new application form for each vacancy a practice manager may decide to have a 'core' form, to which appropriate supplementary questions are added. Alternatively, a standard form can be retained on a word processor and adapted as required.

Supplementary questions can be extremely informative and can be used for every vacancy. It gives the practice an opportunity to seek the applicant's views on a variety of issues. If the practice has a particular weakness that it is anxious to correct or minimize, a supplementary question could be appropriate. For example, the retiring receptionist could be described as the old-fashioned 'dragon' who felt that her sole purpose in life was to prevent patients having access to doctors. The practice needs a complete review of the reception desk and its public image and reputation.

In this situation, supplementary questions would include:

- How do you feel patients should be greeted? Please describe.
- What approach should the receptionist maintain towards patients, and why?
- Should the receptionist get involved in the decision for a patient to see a doctor? Explain reasons.

When the application forms have been returned they can be pre-screened effectively, using the specification as a yardstick. The only deviation from this would be if the most important criterion is 'personality'. There is no substitute for actually meeting the applicants and making a subjective decision about their ability to fit in with the team, if both parties agree that they can work together.

A practice may decide that the ideal number of candidates to offer a first interview is six or eight, with a view to short-list to two or three.

Interviews

These guidelines apply to both first and second interviews. The initial decision is: 'who should interview?' One skilled person is better than any number who do not have a plan or experience. For this reason the practice manager will often be the one to conduct the initial round. For the final interviews others may with to participate, preferably those who will be working most closely with the new person and a partner. However, bear in mind that a selection panel of more than three can be extremely threatening and the candidate may not perform well through 'nerves' alone. The interview needs to be chaired in the same way as any other formal meeting.

The interview must be structured with time allocated to each stage, including an opportunity for the candidate to ask questions and perhaps offer information that was not covered in the application form.

Preparation for interview

- Book an available room.
- Give applicants reasonable warning of the interview date and time.
- Arrange the furniture of the interview room:
  - sun not directly in candidate's eyes.
  - water jug and glasses available.
  - chairs either in a circle or positioned across a (tidy) desk.
- Read the application forms and any supporting information.
- Have a copy of the criteria or specification to hand.
- Ensure that reception staff have a list of appointments and know where to direct candidates.
- Cancel all telephone calls.
- Place a 'do not disturb' sign on the interview room door.
- Brief all members of the interview team immediately prior to interview:
  - who will ask questions, and about what?
  - who will chair the interview?
  - who will make notes?
- Go out and meet each applicant to invite them into the interview room.
- After the interviews, hold a team review:
  - what could have been handled better?
  - who is the preferred candidate?
  - who is the 'first reserve'?
  - nominate a person to write to each candidate, both successful and unsuccessful.
  - keep the applications of very good candidates on file for future reference.

Structure of a 30-minute interview

Minutes	Stages of interview

0   *Introductions and 'warm-up'*
- Introduce all parties.
- Relax the candidate by asking non-threatening questions; eg
  - 'how was your journey?'
  - 'have you been to this medical centre before?'

5   *Explanation*
- Describe the role.
- Ask if there are any queries arising from the application form or job specification.
  - Deal with any questions in full.

10   *General questioning*
- Ask the candidate about previous employment.
- Query any gaps in employment history.
- Ask the candidate to describe her own strengths and weaknesses.
- Why has she applied?
- Why did she leave her last job?
- Always ask open questions to encourage the candidate to talk; ie questions that cannot be answered 'yes' or 'no'.
- Ask questions to match specification to candidate.

20   *Probe*
- Use this time to go back and check any information already received that did not sound quite correct or needs further explanation.

25   *Candidate's questions*
- Allow the candidate to take control of the interview to ask her own questions.
- Listen carefully to any questions; they are an indication of the candidate's views and attitudes.

28   *Ending*

30   Thank the candidate for attending and explain when she can expect to receive a letter or telephone call.

Assessment factors

Positive	Negative
Assured and self-confident	
Unimpeded by nerves	Shy and retiring manner
Comfortable with groups/individuals	Cannot contain anxieties
Has handled people effectively	
Recognizes and uses the strengths of others to achieve objectives	Unable to achieve results by using others
Has worked well as part of a team	
Co-operates with others	Loner
Prepared to compromise	Disruptive
Supportive of team members	Unwilling to contribute to the team
Sensitivity to others	
Approachable	Lacks empathy
Tactful	Lacks tolerance or patience with others
Aware of the implications of situations on others	Superficial appreciation
Has influenced others	
Uses reason and discussion well	Ineffectual in discussion
	Does not use reasoned arguments
Thinks clearly	
Logical	Muddled thinker
Objective	Opinionated
Can distinguish between major and minor issues	Unable to see the wood for the trees
Communicates effectively	
Clear	Confused
Articulate	Verbose
Concise	
Has organized well	
Clear and methodical	Poor delegation
Delegates and follows up well	Does not co-ordinate or follow up
Uses resources effectively	

Positive	Negative
Has a practical approach	
Shows attention to detail	Side-tracked by theory
Realistic	Loses sight of practicalities
Thorough	
Has been decisive	
Uses reason	Avoids or defers decision-making
Uses own judgement	
Gets things done	
Anticipates problems and opportunities	
Keeps an eye on the future	Preoccupied with current
Plans	problems
Identifies future problems and deals with them	Fails to look ahead
Has shown initiative	
Self-motivated	Needs direction
Prepared to lead	Influenced by others
Generates action	
Has set high standards	
Wants to do well	Prepared to accept second best
Sets ambitious, but realistic targets	
Has coped with stress	
Resilient	Panics easily
Calm and unflustered	Thrown by unexpected
Performs well even when under pressure	
Has adapted to change	
Responds positively to new ideas and information	Dogmatic
	Slow to adapt
Reorganizes and re-plans	Resentful
Prepared to work within a system	
Accepts constraints	Reluctant to conform
	Becomes irritated by tasks

References

In the rush to fill a vacancy, references are often forgotten. This is unwise because some people are adept at being interviewed and can deceive the interviewers. The references will, it is hoped, confirm the judgement of the selection team.

It is advisable to take up employment references whenever they are available. These are likely to be unbiased and give an accurate picture of the candidate as an employee. The personal references are almost guaranteed to be good, otherwise they would not have been written on the application form. An example of a reference request is shown in Figure 4.4.

No suitable applicants

If the recruitment process fails to attract the right candidate, it has to be reviewed from the first stage and started again. It will take several weeks to repeat. If all the application forms have been retained, it may be possible to

Standard reference request:

Dear . . . .

Re: [*name and address of candidate*]

The above person has applied for our current vacancy for a

. . . .

Please indicate if you feel the applicant has suitable personal and technical skills to undertake this role effectively.

We would appreciate particular comment on the applicant's reliability, attendance record, punctuality, competence, and ability to protect confidential information.

All information will be treated in strictest confidence, and I can be reached on the above telephone number if you would prefer to provide a verbal reference.

A stamped addressed envelope is provided for your reply.

Thank you for your co-operation.

Figure 4.4:   Example of a standard reference request.

go back to them and re-interview short-listed candidates, or even look again at those that were screened out from the application form.

If insufficient people were attracted, the advertisement and placement could be at fault. This also applies if there were lots of applicants with irrelevant experience.

It is always wise to have a 'first' and 'second' when selecting the successful person. Take up references on both and then, if one falls at the last fence, there is a replacement waiting. This could avoid having to repeat the whole procedure.

Remember that there are only two possible real errors of judgement when recruiting:

1 appointing the wrong person
2 overlooking the right person.

Job descriptions

It is unreasonable to expect that staff will perform their role well unless they have been given a clear outline of their duties and responsibilities. The most effective way of achieving this is via a job description. It has a place in the recruitment process, initial training, appraisal and staff development.

Introducing job descriptions

For existing staff

The people who understand their role in most detail are those actually doing it. If a practice does not have job descriptions and needs to introduce them, staff must be given the opportunity to participate in their formulation. It will reinforce the value and contribution of each member of the team, and could well encourage some self-analysis of performance. In short, the practice has nothing to lose from the exercise.

For new staff

The intended job description may require some minor alteration to take into account any special skills that the successful applicant may have.

A job description should contain the following elements:

- job title
- purpose and objective of the post
- reporting procedure (i.e. who is responsible to whom)

- key elements of the post
- specific tasks
- outline of the internal and external contacts necessary to perform the role.
- any special needs that are not made clear by the job title; eg
  - confidentiality of information
  - specific qualification
- a clause that will allow the staff member to be flexible; eg 'Any duty that may be properly deemed by the partners to be part of the role.'

An outline format of a job description is shown in Figure 4.5.

Contracts of employment

This is one of the main areas of a practice manager's responsibility that requires an understanding of the legal aspects of employment. There are a

Job title: _____
Objective: _____
_____
_____
Responsible to: _____

Key elements:
1
2
3
4
5

Specific tasks:
6
7
8
9
10
11   Any duty that may be properly deemed by the partners as part of the role.

Special requirements:

Figure 4.5: Example of a basic formula for a job description.

variety of laws surrounding the employment of staff, some of which are complex and confusing. The one that probably has the greatest influence is the Employment Protection (Consolidation) Act 1978. This is the one that states that an employer must provide an employee with a written contract of employment by the 13th week of employment, if the employee works more than 16 hours per week.

A practice manager must ensure safe employment procedures, and advice about the legal aspects can be obtained from the FHSA, the British Medical Association, the Advisory, Conciliation and Arbitration Service (ACAS), medical defence organizations and the local job centres. It is essential to keep up to date with the major implications of the current legislation to avoid difficult and costly problems in the future.

We enter into a contractual situation from the moment a verbal job offer is made. This should be confirmed in writing by a formal offer of employment and followed by a contract within the first 13 weeks.

There are standard contract of employment forms available, but some practice managers use their own version that incorporates the main points.

Contents of the contract of employment

- The names and addresses of both parties, ie the employer and the employee.
- Job title.
- Details of the salary structure and any review dates.
- Entitlement to sickness pay.
- How and when salaries are paid.
- Place of employment.
- Hours of work.
- Entitlement to holiday pay.
- Pension arrangements.
- Length of notice to terminate employment.
- Health and safety.
- Disciplinary procedure.
- Grievance procedure.

Other points can be included in addition to, but not instead of, those listed above.

Initial training

We all run on tight staffing levels and every member of staff is required to be operational from day one. A comprehensive initial training period of several weeks may seem to be an unnecessary expense, but it will pay dividends in the long run.

New members of staff will feel welcome if some importance has been attached to their proper introduction to the organization. It will help them to absorb a number of basic facts, that we all take for granted, before the specific work pressures begin in earnest. It will also convey the standards that are achieved and desired. The outline of an initial training programme for a medical secretary is given in Figure 4.6.

The ideal person to monitor the initial training period is a member of staff already performing the new person's role well. She can be assigned to the new person and can advise the practice manager of strengths and weaknesses that emerge during the first few weeks.

It is important that the initial training period remains flexible in both content and duration. Previous experience and the ability to absorb and assimilate information will influence the progress of each individual. The practice manager should have regular, preferably weekly, sessions with the new employee to verify the messages from other staff and to give the individual the opportunity to become involved in her own training.

The initial period should not be confined to the person's future role but should be used to give an understanding of the way the whole organization works.

Appraisal

The word 'appraisal' evokes a number of reactions, almost all of them negative. Handled well, an appraisal system can become a powerful motivating force for staff, especially if there is scope for the individual's salary to be linked to performance.

Many practice managers have been reluctant to introduce an appraisal system, either because they themselves have never experienced it, and therefore have as many concerns as the staff, or because they feel unable to deal with certain disciplinary matters that will inevitably arise and become 'public'. These fears must be overcome to gain all the benefits that appraisals can bring to the practice.

The first step is to decide what the criteria for the various levels of performance will be. These need to be discussed and agreed by the partners before any interviews with staff begin. It is essential that the criteria are then adhered to – that is, the rules are applied fairly to all. It would be naïve to assume that we treat all staff the same; we instinctively find some easier to deal with than others. The appraisal system must eliminate these differences if it is to have any credibility.

Name: _____

Trainer:	Mrs Ann Smith, Medical Secretary
Hours:	8.30 am to 12.30 pm Monday to Friday

Date:	Area:	Attached to:
1.5.94	Introductions to all staff Tour of building	Ann Smith
2.5.94	Conditions of employment Aim of general practice	Practice manager
3.5.94 4.5.94	Appointments system Appointments system	Receptionist Receptionist
5.5.94	Role of reception	Receptionist
8.5.94 9.5.94 10.5.94	Item of service claims Item of service claims Item of service claims	FHSA clerk FHSA clerk FHSA clerk
11.5.94	Health promotion clinics	Receptionist
12.5.94	General administration	Receptionist
	12.00 Progress review	Practice manager
15.5.94	Telephone manner Dealing with complaints	Telephonist, Practice manager
16.5.94	Repeat prescriptions	Receptionist
17.5.94 18.5.94 19.5.94	Medical records and filing Medical records and filing Written communications	Records clerk Records clerk Ann Smith
	12.00 Progress review	Practice manager
22.5.94 to 26.6.94	Attachment to Ann Smith to see role of Medical Secretary	

Figure 4.6: Example of an initial training programme for a medical secretary.

Each practice has a range of ready-made criteria and these should form the basis for setting acceptable standards; for example:

- job descriptions
- practice philosophy on handling patients

- topics covered in staff training sessions
- organizational protocols.

Introducing appraisal

Some public relations work will be necessary to explain why appraisals are going to be introduced. This can be a formal meeting to which all staff are invited or a letter personally addressed to each member of staff (Figure 4.7).

The key word is 'appraisal' and this can be replaced by any number of other descriptions, such as performance review, personnel audit or training assessment. It is also important to explain the degree of staff involvement required if the scheme is to become a two-way exercise rather than a school report type of approach.

Having set the structure it must be followed through, and the interviews should echo the introductory letter and be completed within the given time scale.

Dear [*use name that you would normally use if speaking to the member of staff*]

Over the next few weeks I would like to have an opportunity to have a quiet discussion with you about your role in the medical centre.

The purpose of the interview will be to discuss your current job, identify any future training needs and to have your own views on the way you would like to progress within the team.

Please give these matters some thought, and I would welcome any suggestions or comments you may have to improve our overall efficiency.
When the interviews with all staff have been completed, we will have a clearer idea of the priorities to tackle during the coming year. Your co-operation will be much appreciated.

Yours sincerely,

[*sign with the name by which you are addressed by the staff*]

Practice Manager

Figure 4.7: Sample letter notifying a member of staff of forthcoming appraisal interview.

Structure of appraisal interview

- Always start the interview by asking if the person is clear about its purpose, and deal with any concerns immediately.
- Ask for the person's view of their own performance; eg
  - 'what do you enjoy?'
  - 'what do you find difficult?'
- Guide discussion to analyse strengths and weaknesses.
- Always back up comments with examples, especially when making a criticism.
- Propose ideas for suitable training to correct weaknesses and develop strengths.
- Explore practice and personal issues; eg
  - suitability of hours
  - wish to increase or decrease hours
  - domestic factors that could affect the job.
- Encourage ideas and suggestions by having a free discussion about general issues.
- Summarize key points.
- Congratulate on things done well to end the interview on a high note.

Some practices may transcribe the interview and the comments on to a standard form; this can be drawn up before, during or after the interview. To be effective, the form needs to be simple and flexible – that is, not too many specific issues. A copy of the appraisal summary should be handed to the member of staff and another filed for future reference. The following year's appraisal can be compared to the preceding one to monitor progress.

Team building

The practice manager has a strong obligation to the team, and a sensible manager invests time and effort to strengthen the team at every opportunity.

Building a team, and maintaining it, incorporates all the skills required of a good personnel manager. Some techniques can be learned; others require personal qualities that either we have or we must find ways to compensate. For example, we cannot learn to be sensitive, but we can take advice from a discreet and reliable member of the team before introducing something new.

There are some simple guidelines that will protect the practice manager from the obvious pitfalls, some of which have been covered already in previous text and will be mentioned only briefly here.

Team building has four main ingredients:

- motivation
- communication
- accountability
- equality.

Motivation

Before we can begin to build a team we must break it down into each component part, that is the individuals concerned. Each one will have a different personality, different standards and a different reason for working. All of these need to be analysed and then a plan formulated to deal with them. Much of this ground will have been covered by the appraisal interview, and each member of staff should have a clear image of his or her place within the organization.

There are a number of motivating factors, and the following are based on Abraham Maslow's hierarchy of seven human needs,

1 Physiological – food, water, temperature control.
2 Safety – security, freedom from threat.
3 Social – love, affiliation, acceptance by others.
4 Esteem – prestige, status, self-esteem, respect from others.
5 Cognitive – knowledge, understanding, curiosity.
6 Aesthetic – beauty, art, structure.
7 Self-fulfilment – achievement, realization of potential.

Maslow ranked 1 as the most important and 7 as the least, although they are all interrelated. What motivates individuals depends upon what they already have and what they want. A person working solely to feed the family is unlikely to be too concerned about the social life offered by the practice. Conversely, a person who wants to avoid the boredom of staying at home with no financial pressure to work is likely to be interested in the social aspects. The wise practice manager will know the staff well enough to know which approach is most likely to gain agreement from each individual, and use it to full advantage.

Communication

The level of information required by each member of the team is often divided into the 'need to know' and the 'nice to know'.

- 'Need to know' – information that is centred purely on the task and confined to the skills necessary to perform effectively.

- 'Nice to know' – information about general topics that are indirectly related to the task and items that are intended to stimulate thought about all aspects of the organization.

Ideally, each and every team member will need a combination of both to have specific information about their personal role and an indication of the broader issues that they should be working towards.

Communication is such an important topic that it merits a complete chapter later in the book that should be read in conjunction with this section.

Accountability

To feel part of any team we must have clearly defined objectives and responsibilities. This makes us both individual and important in our contribution to the whole. Job descriptions, training and appraisals are fundamental to the process of accountability.

The other advantage of accountability is the reassurance that a manager can trace back problems to their source, and deal with them accordingly. It is very frustrating when trying to follow through a problem to find that all the staff blame everyone else. This cannot happen with defined responsibilities and a clear reporting structure (Figure 4.8).

Accountability will also engender a sense of pride in work done well. This in turn will improve and maintain higher standards.

Counselling

So far we have looked at the ways that a practice manager can increase the efficiency of the practice by improving staff performance. However, there are times when we must cease to be 'the boss' and become a friend. It would be naïve to assume that domestic issues can be kept away from work. As a general rule, a manager will prompt a discussion about such problems only

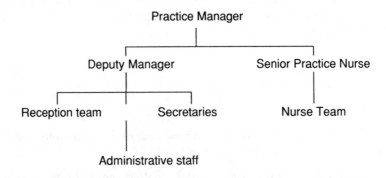

Figure 4.8: A practice hierarchy/reporting structure.

if the individual's performance or attendance is affected. A practice manager must maintain a sensible balance between maintaining her authority and being an approachable human being. If the relationships are correct the staff will come to the manager with a domestic problem before it becomes a disciplinary type of discussion.

Counselling is a skill that needs to be learned if it is to be done well. There are many courses available and a practice manager should try to attend at least one during a career, preferably sooner than later.

Such conversations often arise during appraisal interviews, either because the atmosphere is conducive for staff to divulge confidential information about their home life or in response to a criticism about something routine, such as time keeping.

The key to effective counselling is listening and pointing out the individuals' options. It is never a piece of home-spun advice that starts 'If I were you I would do . . .'. Our own feelings must be hidden, especially a horrified reaction to a piece of personal information. The aim is to offer individuals an opportunity to explore their own feelings and decide their own course of action.

The practice manager must be clear about her own personal capabilities and be aware that, in certain cases, more expert help is needed. We are ideally placed to suggest that the GP be consulted, and we have information about professional counsellors and self-help groups. It is sheer arrogance to assume that we can solve every problem in a person's life – we can't. What we can do is offer to make short-term compromises at work, possibly a period of unpaid leave or an alteration to working hours. We also reassure the individual that they can talk freely to someone who shows empathy with their circumstances.

Personnel records

A personnel file, however simple, should be maintained for each member of staff. These may not seem necessary when things are going well, but they are invaluable when things go wrong. Fortunately, very few practices have undergone the trauma of an Industrial Tribunal and had to prove that it has acted fairly and reasonably, and followed its own employment policies. This is the worst possible scenario, but it can be a real danger when a practice manager deals with a situation badly. Staff are fully aware that they have rights under various employment laws, and they can access this information very easily if they wish to. Such an occurrence can be prevented by following sound personnel procedures like those described in this chapter. However, following them is not enough and they must be recorded accurately.

Contents of a personnel file

- Application form.
- References.
- Letter of appointment.
- Copy of contract.
- Copy of each appraisal.
- Record of significant discussions.
- Record of any changes to working hours.
- Promotions or demotions.

In addition, there should be a method of recording absence and holidays for all staff, and a means of recording all training sessions and attendees. These details can be effectively kept in a diary used exclusively for that purpose.

Access to a personnel file should be given only to the individual, never to a third party. In this respect, personnel files should be treated with the same code of confidentiality as a patient's medical record.

Disciplinary procedures

As previously mentioned, each employment contract must include a statement about the disciplinary process and the grievance procedure.

Each step in the disciplinary process must be fair both to the employer and to the individual, from the first informal discussion to, if necessary, the dismissal. Handled correctly, many situations are resolved in the early stages because the member of staff had not realized the problem until it was brought to her attention or because of the opportunity for additional training. Very few situations need to reach a dismissal.

Employees must be made aware of the issues that could endanger their performance and have the disciplinary steps defined in writing.

Disciplinary matters can usually be divided into four groups: gross breaches of regulations, misconduct, standards of work and criminal acts outside work.

Gross breaches of regulations

Examples of a gross breach of regulations include:

- breach of confidentiality
- mishandling of practice funds or property
- falsification of expenses
- failure to obey smoking policies.

Summary or instant dismissal

Certain breaches of regulations may result in summary or instant dismissal; for example, disclosing confidential information to a third party. Be warned: an employee could be deemed to have been dismissed unfairly if no opportunity was given to explain her actions. Be particularly careful where information has been given by another person and fully investigate each instance before taking any action. If it is inappropriate for the employee to continue working during such an investigation, she can be suspended on full pay. Employees should be given the opportunity to be accompanied at any disciplinary interview.

Misconduct

Examples of misconduct include:

- poor timekeeping
- unacceptable absence
- appearance not meeting the required standard
- poor relationships with other members of staff
- unacceptable personal behaviour.

Standards of work

This area is self-explanatory and relates to failures to meet the standards required in the job description and those set in training sessions.

Criminal acts outside work

If the practice learns than an employee has been found guilty of a criminal act, it may have a bearing on that person's continued employment; for example, drug offences. Each instance must be fully investigated before taking action.

Disciplinary process

The process can be stopped at any stage, if the employee demonstrates that she has reached the required standard. A suitable length of time must be allowed between each step for the employee to put right any criticisms, and it is good practice to fix the date of the subsequent interview. Even if the process can be halted, it will give the practice manager an opportunity to confirm that the necessary standards have been reached.

Step 1   Informal discussion with practice manager.

Step 2   Verbal discussion with practice manager.
             Arrange retraining, if appropriate.

From this point the employee must be given the opportunity to be accompanied.

Step 3   Formal discussion with practice manager.
             Written summary of criticisms, a copy of which must be given to employee.
             Arrange further retraining, if appropriate.

Step 4   Formal interview with practice manager and a partner.
             A warning of dismissal will be given should there be any future incident, or failure to reach the required standard.

             A letter summarizing the interview must be sent or handed to the employee. Receipt of this letter must be acknowledged.

Step 5   An interview with the practice manager and a partner.
             Dismissal.

             A detailed account of the interview should be written and held on file.
             The employee can ask for a letter stating reasons for dismissal.

Appeals

At the outset of the disciplinary process the employee must be made aware of the appeal procedure, to be used if she feels that she has been unfairly treated. If the practice manager has dealt with the situation, a panel of partners should constitute the appeal committee. The final level of appeal is the full partnership.

Grievance procedure

The contract of employment must contain a grievance procedure. This is the mechanism by which an employee can complain against unfair or improper treatment.
   A typical grievance procedure would read as follows:

Problems and misunderstandings arise from time to time, whenever a group of people work together. We prefer such situations to be discussed openly and dealt with quickly. If you have a complaint or grievance, please discuss it with your immediate superior or the practice manager. If you feel unable to approach either of these people, then any partner can be approached.

The practice undertakes to investigate any such complaints and to keep the employee informed of their views, after suitable deliberations.

Leaving the practice

Resignations

When an employee wishes to leave, she should be asked to place her resignation in writing, preferably giving her reasons. This should then be filed with the personnel file. An employee is required to give at least one week's notice if she has been employed for one month or longer. If the contract of employment gives a longer period of notice, for example one month, the longer period applies. Employees should be encouraged to give as much notice as possible to allow the practice manager to make plans for recruitment or staff restructure.

Termination of employment

The standard scale of notice than an employer is required to give an employee is:

Continuous employment	Minimum notice
More than 1 months but less than 2 years	1 week
For 2 years	2 weeks
More than 2 years	At least 1 week for each completed year to a maximum of 12 weeks

This requirement does not apply when:

- the employee normally works fewer than 16 hours per week, unless that employment has been continuous for at least 5 years for at least 8 hours per week
- the employee is on a fixed-term contract.

Personnel development

Practice management is an evolving role and there is evidence of a career structure. Instead of staying with one practice for life, there are opportunities to move into fund management, business management in hospitals and senior jobs in the FHSA, not to mention a move to larger practices or consortia.

In view of the ever-changing nature of the job, practice managers need to enhance and increase their skills whenever possible. Most partners have an agreement about a suitable (and desirable) amount of study leave that can be taken in addition to holiday each year. There is no reason why practice managers should not negotiate a similar arrangement for themselves.

There are a range of courses available from professional health bodies, management colleges and business consultants. All managers should do their own assessment of personal strengths and weaknesses and prioritize the training they need. Often the FHSA will be willing to consider setting up a particular seminar if there is enough demand, and the Training Officer at the FHSA is a good contact to cultivate. Other practice managers may be willing to offer a short working attachment on a reciprocal basis. One can always learn from the methods and systems in place elsewhere, and become more professional in the process.

Practice manager groups

When things go badly in a practice and we seem to have been on the receiving end of everyone else's problems, it is easy to feel a sense of frustration and isolation. This can be combated by approaching other practice managers or joining a recognized group. The main official body is the Association of Health Centre and Practice Administrators (AHCPA). There is also the Association of Medical Secretaries, Practice Administrators and Receptionists (AMSPAR), but this might be particularly suitable for the practice staff.

There are also many unofficial groups around the country that perform an equally valuable function. This type of peer group contact is essential, if only for reassurance that we are not alone and that our difficulties are often shared by others. The groups usually meet regularly, ideally during the working day, on an informal basis. It is not necessary to have officers, agendas and minutes; the main purpose is mutual support and the ability to discuss issues with a group who understand the diverse demands made of the practice manager. If there is not such a group in your area, why not start one?

5 Training and the Primary Care Team

Why train?

UNTIL 30 years ago most doctors entering general practice were shown an empty consulting room, a full waiting room and told to get on with it! It was assumed that hospital experience and basic medical training were sufficient. However, the idea that medicine in the community was in some way different from hospital practice was just beginning to take root. Training for general practice was in its infancy.

The new receptionist fared only slightly better. 'Sitting with Nellie' was the accepted, indeed the only, method of training staff. 'Nellie' told her what to do, showed her how to do it and, after a couple of weeks, left her to discover the rest for herself! The title of practice manager was practically unknown.

Both doctors and receptionists learned fast, no doubt acquiring good habits as well as bad. The necessary knowledge and skills to do the job were picked up by trial and error, and some very inappropriate attitudes were acquired along the way. For example, GPs aimed for an average consulting time of six minutes, and receptionists soon accepted their role as 'dragon at the gate'. The idea of the practice team had yet to be conceived.

Over the years, as the importance of general practice within the health service increased, the primary health care team developed into a complex matrix organization. However, until recently, the methods of training within that organization have failed to keep pace.

It is now generally accepted that quality of care and job satisfaction go hand in hand. Contented staff need to know not only what they are doing but also why they are doing it. They must understand how their individual jobs contribute to the care of the patients and the smooth running of the practice team. Nowadays they need not only to be trained but also to continue their education and personal development in order to keep up to date.

This chapter aims to:

- outline some educational concepts in relation to primary care
- discuss ways in which the educational needs of teams and individuals can be identified
- explore the methods of learning and teaching available

- describe the educational networks that presently exist within the health service
- identify the skills and resources required to plan and manage the educational activities of a practice.

An educational environment

People are the most valuable resource of any practice. They deserve the optimum by way of training in order to achieve their maximum potential.

What factors help to create a productive educational environment?

Relationships
Democratic relationships create a co-operative atmosphere.

Knowledge
Activity is a natural consequence when people are given facts, but when there is a lack of information the consequent anxiety breeds uncertainty and enthusiasm is lost.

Support
Clear instructions not only improve confidence but also generate excitement and satisfaction.

Form
A structured programme of education gives a feeling of security and importance – a feeling of belonging to the organization.

Needs
Identifying a person's needs and potential and taking these into account within the constraints of the job results in increased job satisfaction and enhanced motivation.

Education improves motivation, commitment and therefore the quality of care.

Training practice staff

Initial assessment and induction training

Initial assessment should really be part of the selection procedure before employment. The pre-employment interview should ask the following questions.

- What knowledge and skills does the applicant have as a result of past experience?
- Is the applicant flexible enough to fit into the practice team?
- Are the applicant's attitudes appropriate and, if not, can they be modified by training and experience?

All new staff, and those receiving promotion, should undergo induction training. Details of how this may be achieved are given in Chapter 4. Appraisal continues during this induction period and is a two-way process – the employee learning the details of the new job, and the employer discovering the level of the new person's knowledge and capabilities. By the end of the probationary period the employer should have a good idea of the new employee's educational needs and work potential.

This information should be shared at an informal appraisal session. Strengths and weaknesses should be agreed, and targets set for future training and achievements. Training thus becomes an integral part of performance review and personal appraisal, and is accepted as a natural and constructive part of practice life.

Setting up a staff training programme

Planning a staff training programme must take account of information about the following.

1 What the employer believes that staff need in order to improve performance and satisfaction in their daily work.
2 What new skills and knowledge they need to acquire in order to cope with future planned developments.
3 What the staff themselves feel they need/would like to know in order to expand their horizons.

This information is derived from a knowledge of the practice business plan, as described in Chapter 3, and an educational appraisal.

The educational appraisal

All staff should have the opportunity of being appraised (Chapter 4). An assessment of the educational needs, not only of individuals but also of the whole team, should emerge from this process. Discussion during the appraisal interview should provide answers to the following questions.

- What aspects of work are enjoyed most?
- Are these the aspects that they feel they do well? If so, can they explain why?

- Would they, as part of the educational programme, be prepared to explain to others how they carry out that part of their work?
- Which parts of work do they actively dislike and try to avoid? Why?
- How might these aspects be made more interesting?
- What in the present job would they like to do that they are not doing at present?
- Have they any personal ambitions for the future?

The answers to these questions will contribute to the formation of an educational plan for individual members of staff as well as for the whole team.

Knowledge of the resources available for training

The resources one must have available in order to undertake training are time, talent, outside agencies and money.

Time

Time is perhaps the most difficult commodity to negotiate. Partnerships vary in their commitment to training and, unless care is taken, the pressure of work will erode the time set aside and interruptions will further detract from the effectiveness of educational sessions. It is essential that not only is sufficient time set aside each week for staff training but also that the time is 'protected'. Ideally, all the staff should be able to attend. Many practices choose to close the surgery for about an hour each week in order that the training session can take place uninterrupted and, provided this fact is well advertised and an efficient emergency system is in operation, patients accept this without complaint.

Talent

'In-house' resources
Many meetings can be run by the staff themselves. Extremely effective sessions can be held on such mundane subjects as:

- filing procedures – how to find missing notes!
- how to load the photocopier with paper
- how to 'back-up' the computer before switching off, or carry out simple searches.

Doctors, practice and community nurses and health visitors are often only too pleased to make informal presentations on, for example:

- the practice diabetic or asthma clinic

- family planning
- obstetrics or child health surveillance.

These sessions are particularly effective when the results of some 'in-practice' audit can be included. This will not only show what is being achieved but also promote discussion which may further improve co-operation and performance.

External speakers
Outside speakers with particular expertise can be invited to address members of the primary health care team on subjects of particular interest. Sessions of this type lend themselves to interdisciplinary learning. For example, the local ambulance service might be asked to train the whole practice team in the first aid procedures for cardio-pulmonary resuscitation. The fact that doctors, staff and other team members all carry out this training together can be a rewarding experience and a very good team-building exercise.

Outside agencies

Courses for receptionists
Many organizations now run courses of this type. They vary in quality and content according to the interests of the responsible organization. Information about what is available in your area may be obtained from the local:

- Family Health Services Authority's (FHSA) training manager
- members of the Association of Health Centre and Practice Administrators (AHCPA) or Association of Medical Secretaries, Practice Administrators and Receptionists (AMSPAR)
- colleges of further education
- postgraduate medical centre administrator
- practice managers.

Sometimes local practice managers get together to form a support group and arrange their own extended courses for receptionists.

Practice managers
Practice managers also need to develop their management skills and keep up to date. A number of specialized courses now exist to cater for this need and, in addition to the above agencies, it may be worth while contacting the Association of Medical Secretaries, Practice Administrators and Receptionists (AMSPAR).

Practice nurse training
On the whole, practice nurses see themselves as accountable to the doctors of the practice but, as practice employees, their training and education are often administered by the practice manager. These days practice nurses are

taking increasing responsibility for disease prevention, health education and the care of patients with such chronic diseases as diabetes, asthma and hypertension. As a result, they require special training in order to learn new skills and keep up to date.

In some areas, practice nurses can learn with and from doctors. Within the practice this usually takes the form of the joint production of disease management protocols, whilst elsewhere most postgraduate medical centres now welcome practice nurses to practically all clinical meetings designed for GPs. The time may soon come when practice nurses have to produce evidence of continuing education in the same way as their general practitioner employers.

However, not all nurse education can be shared with doctors. Practice nurses need to develop skills of their own, and special courses are now run by many postgraduate centres, university departments and colleges of further education which cater particularly for their needs.

Facilitators

Facilitators now exist in most Health Service regions. They are experienced nurses and doctors whose job is to promote practice activities in health care and medical audit. They are employed either by the FHSA – in which case they are likely to be responsible to the Medical Audit Advisory Group (MAAG) – or the District Health Authority (DHA). Some nurse facilitators have a particular remit; for example, to assist practices in the setting up of health education programmes and 'well person' clinics.

Because education and practice development go hand in hand, facilitators are invariably willing to co-operate in practice training programmes. As 'outsiders' they have the great advantage of being able to talk to all members of the practice team in an unbiased way, and thus stimulate an atmosphere of understanding and co-operation.

Budgets

Most practices now recognize the importance of training, and set money aside to pay for it. To encourage this, FHSAs now allocate funds to each practice for training purposes as part of their total staff budget. This money is earmarked for training but can be spent by the practice according to its own educational priorities. Whilst this method of reimbursement for staff training may limit the amount that can be done, it does not prevent the practice from putting in a bid for special training. Provided that funds are available and it can be shown that patient care is likely to improve as a result, the request is likely to succeed.

Vocational training for general practice

After qualification, doctors must spend a year working as house officers in hospital before becoming fully registered. Only then can they begin the three years of vocational training required by law to become principals in general practice.

Vocational training for general practice consists of two years in recognized hospital jobs (such as paediatrics, obstetrics, gynaecology, psychiatry, accident and emergency, and geriatrics) and a third year in an approved training practice.

There are two ways in which doctors can undergo training. They may either design their own 'scheme' by applying for hospital jobs and a training practice of their own choosing, or they can join a vocational training scheme based on a district general hospital. These schemes guarantee proper experience in approved posts all within the same district, thus allowing participants to remain in one area for the three years of their training.

Vocational training schemes are run by one or more local course organizers, who are responsible for the 'trainees' during their time on the scheme. A number of training practices are attached to each scheme, and one of the partners, having gone through a training and selection process, is approved as trainer (*see* 'Vocational training for general practice', later).

These experienced GPs act as a personal tutor for the trainees while they are in the training practices. During this time the trainees work as a member of the partnership and learn as much as possible about the intricacies of primary care. This is achieved by treating patients and by a series of tutorials. Trainees also take part in an educational programme outside the practice which involves their release from practice from time to time.

Although trainees have a service commitment to the training practice, their position is technically supernumerary. The time spent by the trainers and other members of the partnership in teaching is balanced by the amount of work done by the trainee.

Whilst trainers are responsible for organizing the trainees' educational programme within the practice, other members of the primary health care team have become more involved, as interdisciplinary learning and teamwork have increasingly been recognized as important. Practice managers therefore play an important part in vocational training.

1 They are responsible for the contractual arrangements of training. (Although vocational trainees are employed by the practice, their salary is reimbursed by the FHSA.)
2 Under the trainers' supervision, they organize the trainees' work within the practice and set aside protected time for the training programme.
3 They often contribute to the teaching themselves. Practice managers' skills and knowledge in such areas as finance, teamwork, employment, admin-

istration and planning are an invaluable part of any vocational training curriculum.

Students

Medical students

These days most medical schools arrange for students to spend some time in general practice. The amount of time set aside for this can vary from two to six weeks, and requires organization.

Student health visitors and nurses

Increasingly, other disciplines are making the experience of work in the community an integral part of training. Students of health visiting, community nursing and midwifery are, from time to time, placed under the supervision of 'practical work teachers', who are experienced members of primary health care teams.

Interdisciplinary learning

The presence of students and doctors in vocational training produces a very stimulating atmosphere. Learners have a habit of asking awkward questions and constantly challenge accepted ideas. In responding, those involved in training have constantly to organize their thoughts and justify their actions. This often produces new ideas that improve patient care. Opportunities for joint learning and teaching also exist and these offer great educational possibilities, but require careful planning.

The practice manager is in a good position to promote and co-ordinate these activities. For example, a standard programme can be developed for introducing students to the work of the primary health care team. Such a programme can form a useful part of the induction process of all members of the primary health care team by improving 'role perception' and teamwork. Whilst the programme itself will need to be adapted for individual needs, it is likely to contain some or all of the following elements.

- Sitting in the waiting room and talking informally to patients in order to gain insight into their concerns and expectations.
- Answering the telephone in reception and working alongside an experienced receptionist.

- Spending time with health visitors and community nurses, and attending the various clinics run both in and out of the practice.
- 'Sitting in' with doctors in order to gain insight into their individual working patterns.
- Spending time with other agencies, such as the local chemist, social work department and funeral director.
- Interviewing patients in their homes after a surgery or home visit by one of the team, in order to gain insight into their concerns and expectations.

As many of the above require the co-operation of patients, it is important that proper consent is obtained and strict confidentiality maintained. Patients attending surgeries must be informed of the practice's involvement with training. It is a good idea to put up a notice to that effect. Patients must also be informed when students are likely to be present. This is best done by receptionists giving patients a leaflet when they arrive and explaining that, if they have any reservations about a third party being present during their consultation, the student will withdraw.

Experience has shown that most people appreciate the need for training and are only too willing to co-operate. Word of the practice's involvement in training soon gets around and most patients believe that, as a result, they receive a higher standard of care than they might otherwise expect.

Continuing medical education

General practitioners, like all professionals, have to keep up to date and acquire new skills. Most doctors continue their education out of interest and enthusiasm for their work, but the government also encourages GPs to do so by paying the Postgraduate Education Allowance (PGEA) to all those who fulfil certain criteria. To qualify for this payment, GPs must produce evidence of having attended an average of 15 days' postgraduate education over a period of three years – five days in each of three areas:

- disease management
- health education and prevention
- service management.

Certificates of attendance at approved meetings are supplied by the organizers, and many practice managers oversee the arrangements for payment of the allowance on behalf of the doctors in their practice. The paperwork is submitted to the FHSA, who then make payments on a quarterly basis.

Partnerships vary in the way in which this allowance is shared, and the method is usually stated in a clause in the partnership agreement. The most usual arrangement is for the money to go directly to the partner who qualified for it. Thus, if a doctor chooses not to fulfil his educational responsibilities in any given period, the partnership, as a whole, does not suffer. If, because of illness or some other good reason, a doctor falls behind with his accreditation, there are rules which, within limits, allow him to 'catch up' without penalty. On the whole, however, most GPs have no difficulty in fulfilling the requirements.

Educational organizations

Like everything else in the health service, the organizational structure of postgraduate education for doctors has undergone considerable change in the last few years. What follows is a brief description of how things are organized at present. (*See also* Fig. 5.1.)

At a regional level, the Postgraduate Dean, now called the Director of Postgraduate Medical Education/Training, is, in theory, responsible for all postgraduate education, whether it takes place in hospital or the community. The post is usually a university appointment and the incumbent works with the Regional Health Authority and a number of regional advisers (one for each specialty). Together with others they form the Regional Education Committee.

The Regional Adviser in General Practice, a member of the above committee, works with his own General Practice Subcommittee to administer postgraduate education in the two areas of vocational training and continuing medical education.

Vocational training for general practice

Most vocational training schemes are based on district general hospitals and postgraduate medical centres. The schemes are administered by course organizers, who are GPs with a special interest in education. They are appointed by the General Practitioner Subcommittee and responsible to the Regional Adviser in General Practice.

The approval of training practices is the responsibility of the Regional Adviser and the General Practitioner Subcommittee. Before approval, GP trainers usually have to undertake some form of training in teaching methods, and the practice itself is normally evaluated by a visit from the authorities in order to assess its suitability for training.

Whilst the mechanisms for approval may vary from region to region, they all conform to a set of national standards laid down by the Joint Committee for Postgraduate Training in General Practice (JCPTGP). From time to time, representatives of the JCPTGP visit the regions to see that the standards are being applied.

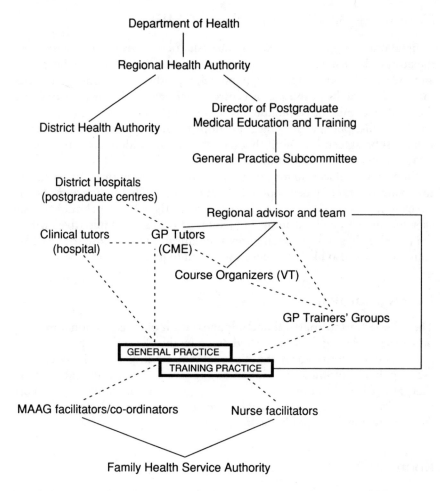

Figure 5.1: Educational networks. Dotted lines mark lines of influence; solid lines show lines of accountability.

Doctors undergoing general practice training are technically employees of the practice and require a contract of employment. The local vocational training scheme may have its own standard contract but more than likely it will not, in which case the British Medical Association are happy to send a sample document to members on request. It is usual for practice managers to administer these aspects of training.

Doctors who have successfully completed vocational training are issued with a certificate qualifying them to enter into contract with an FHSA and become a principal in general practice. Details of how this is administered can be obtained from local course organizers or the regional office.

Continuing Medical Education (CME)

General practice tutors now exist in most districts. They usually work from the postgraduate medical centres attached to most district general hospitals, and their job involves organizing, and helping others to organize, meetings for GPs, both in the postgraduate centre and elsewhere. Many are extending their influence into the community by promoting 'in practice', 'inter-practice' and 'inter-disciplinary' meetings. It is hoped that a national job description will soon be agreed but, until this takes place, the wide variations in local CME arrangements will continue.

'In-practice' education for doctors and all members of the primary health care team is a rapidly developing field and one in which practice managers have an important part to play. In this context the GP tutor should be seen as someone who will encourage and support educational initiatives within the practice. The link between audit and education is so close that MAAG facilitators are also likely to be well disposed to give help and advice.

PGEA approval

The criteria for the approval and administration of an educational meeting under the PGEA regulations are laid down by the General Practice Subcommittee and administered by the Regional Adviser in General Practice. Any meeting that fulfils these criteria can be approved, and educational meetings that take place within the practice are recognized in the same way as those in postgraduate centres. Details of how to apply for approval can be obtained from the regional postgraduate office.

Sponsorship

Many agencies, particularly the pharmaceutical industry, have resources available for training. Apart from straightforward financial support, they can often offer films, videotapes, workbooks and other literature – even interactive computer programs. Many of them are excellent but care must be taken to ensure that they are relevant to primary care and that they do not contain promotional material, otherwise they cannot be approved for PGEA. If there is any doubt, the local GP tutor should be consulted.

Summary

Practice managers have a crucial role to play in the educational activities of general practice, not only because of their organizational and management skills but also because of the unique position they hold within the primary health care team.

Education can take place in many different ways and cover many different fields of activity within the life of a practice. The ways in which a practice manager can be involved in and influence education within primary care have been described in the earlier parts of this chapter. They may be summarized by remembering the mnemonic 'FAME' and giving two functions to each letter of the word.

Facilitation	Appraisal	Management	Education
Finance	Administration	Meetings	Evaluation

Facilitation

By fostering an atmosphere in which education is accepted as a normal part of practice life, the practice manager will improve job satisfaction and the overall quality of care.

Finance

Education costs money. The training budget must be managed, the financial arrangements of PGEA require administration and, when the practice is involved in vocational training, the trainee has to be paid!

Appraisal

People change and organizations develop. Education is an integral part of this process and should include a system of individual appraisal that will identify the educational needs of the practice.

Administration

Training activities require oversight. Systems have to be designed, programmes published and proper records maintained.

Management

Whilst administration is concerned mainly with processes and resources, management is more about people – how they are affected by change, how they carry out their work, and how they acquire the knowledge and skills to remain effective members of the practice team.

Meetings

Quite apart from getting people together for educational sessions, the pro-grammes themselves require co-operative planning. Meetings are an efficient way of achieving this task.

Education

Practice managers should not neglect their own education. Local support groups and visits to other practices can be of great value, and there are an increasing number of specialized courses available.

Most practice managers now have a teaching role within the practice. They have a great deal of expertise in finance, administration and management which they can share with doctors (especially vocational trainees) and other members of staff.

Evaluation

Evaluation is an essential part of any educational process. It forms the beginning and the end of the educational cycle. The process draws on both appraisal and audit, and helps to determine the effectiveness of past edu-cational activities and define the future curriculum.

Without training the continuing development of any practice will suffer. Training promotes confidence, job satisfaction and a sense of worth which results in true teamwork and improved quality of care.

This chapter has discussed the importance of continuing education for all members of the primary health care team and underlined the essential role played by the practice manager.

Further reading

Priority Objectives for General Practice Vocational Training. Occasional Paper No 30. Royal College of General Practitioners, London

Working Together, Learning Together. Occasional Paper No 33. Royal College of General Practitioners, London.

For reference

The Statement of Fees and Allowances.

Training for General Practice. Joint Committee for Postgraduate Training in General Practice, 14 Princes Gate, London SW7 1PU.

6 Communication

In this chapter we consider what is involved when we talk about communication. This can be approached on two levels: interpersonal communication and communication systems.

'Communication' is the ability to impart information, knowledge and ideas from one person to another, either individually or in groups. It forms the framework without which organizations will fail to function.

We all feel that we can express ourselves in speech, and because of this there is often a failure to grasp the complex nature of communication that must exist even in quite small organizations. Communication may be simply broken down into:

- collection of information from the periphery to the centre
- transmission of instructions from the centre to the periphery
- interactive communication in pairs or groups – this may be formal or informal.

These aspects of communication are involved in:

- formation of policy
- resolution of problems and conflict
- training and instruction.

Communication is a two-way process. It involves listening and receiving as well as imparting information and feelings. It is a dynamic process with subtle nuances. Even listening is a dynamic process, involving eye contact and making encouraging gestures and sounds. Body language can often say more than the spoken word; for example, if the person to whom you are talking looks at you and leans slightly forward, this indicates to you that he is receptive. If, however, his eyes are roaming away from your face and he is leaning back in his chair, this probably indicates the opposite response.

Good communication is essential for a practice manager, but how is it achieved? Much depends on personality and the ability to overcome barriers. Practice managers need the ability to communicate freely with busy, individualistic doctors whilst, equally, they need to have an easy relationship with subordinates or members of the attached staff such as health visitors or community nurses. Doctors are often seen to be powerful figures but the skill and knowledge of the practice manager comprise a source of power upon which others rely. If a manager is sensitive to this status barrier to communication, she will be more approachable to her juniors who might otherwise be in awe of her.

Methods of communication

The main methods of communication are:

- the spoken word
- the written word and pictures
- using the telephone (including answering machines), facsimile, computers, modems, VDUs and videos as well as printed matter.

The spoken word

This is the most sophisticated means of communication and includes non-verbal behaviour. The spoken word is essential for group activity and allows maximum deployment of personalities.

Essential factors

- Sensitivity and awareness.
- Ability to see things from the other person's point of view.
- Accessibility for face-to-face communication in private.
- Ability to listen and understand and to be understood.

Written communication

This is essential for the recording of facts – for example, agreements, contracts, minutes, records, letters and telephone messages. The language used must be clear and easily understood, and yet concise. Poor use of language makes the meaning opaque or even ambiguous. The disadvantage of written communication is that it is not face to face.

Internal and external communication

Written messages – internal

How can the practice manager design a fail-safe system so that urgent messages do not get lost and are acted upon appropriately? A practice policy can require that all messages include the name of the person taking the message, the date and the time of the message and to whom the message is directed. Making individuals responsible for their recording is more likely to produce messages that are well written and clear.

Day book – internal

This is a book in which every message is recorded, together with:

- the date and time it was taken
- who it is from
- who it is for
- who took the message.

The message should be ticked when it has been seen. All members of staff should check the book regularly, before leaving the building and upon their return. The advantage of this method of communication is that there is a permanent record, which may be valuable if anything goes wrong.

Memorandum – internal

It is helpful to use a proforma (Figure 6.1), which will have several headings. The initials of every member of staff should be included, and may be ticked by the relevant individuals to confirm receipt of the memorandum.

```
                    Lee Bank Group Practice

   To: _____

   From: _____

   Date: _____

   Message: _____


                              Initials: _____
```

Figure 6.1:   Example of headings for a memorandum form.

Notice boards – internal or external

These should be located where they are easily seen – at the correct height – readily accessible to those who are expected to see the notices. For example, it is unlikely that members of staff will read a notice board if they do not normally pass by it during their working day.

A member of staff should be given the responsibility of updating the board regularly and displaying up-to-date relevant information. A 'Keep warm in winter' poster is out of place on a hot sunny day in the middle of summer.

White boards – internal or external

Some practices use notices written on white boards to inform patients which doctor is on call for the day or if a particular doctor is running late.

Moving message displays – external

This system of communication is versatile and space saving. A variety of information may be displayed and stored for recall at a later date. Messages may be 'inviting' – for example, in the autumn patients can be informed of the availability of 'flu vaccinations; or they may be informative – for example, giving a health promotion message or even welcoming and light-hearted if appropriate.

Newsletters – internal or external

Some practices produce their own newsletter, which gives them the opportunity to tell patients about new projects or innovations that might be taking place behind the scenes. They may also be used to invite patients to make suggestions or comments about the practice.

A newsletter produced for communication within an organization can help to confirm the practice identity and make it easier for part-time staff to feel that they belong. It can also help a new member of staff, coming as a stranger into a closely knit community, to get a feel of how the practice performs.

Posters, leaflets, notices – internal or external

There is certainly no shortage of paper to display in the waiting room; the difficulty is in deciding what *not* to put in that last available space. Practice managers should encourage one member of staff to take responsibility for posters and leaflets, with perhaps one of the doctors overseeing health messages that the practice wishes to support. It is an important task that should receive an adequate time slot.

Annual report – external

Practices are requested to produce an annual report in which they record certain activities undertaken during the previous year. It is worth mentioning here that, although this may initially appear to be an onerous task, for practices that are already recording so much data, it should be used to provide a strategy for the future. By identifying objectives, it can set targets for the following year. FHSAs provide guidelines for practices prior to the date of submission of the report.

Protocols – internal or external

Since the introduction of the government's new contract for GPs practices have been asked to provide protocols for a variety of activities, an example of this being the provision of health promotion services to patients. Practices applying for Band 3 Health Promotion and Chronic Disease Management have had to submit protocols prior to being accepted by the FHSA. When setting standards of quality, it is essential to have protocols that are clear, but concise, to enable team members performing the task to achieve objectives.

Communications with hospitals, FHSAs, health authorities, etc

The most-used method of written communication is still by letter, and for this reason it is worth while taking a little extra time to maintain a high standard of letter writing.

Many doctors take for granted their in-depth knowledge of medical terminology, and it is up to the practice manager to encourage them to be clear and articulate in their dictating. In the same way, it is vital that practice managers check that their secretaries have a high standard of typing and presentation. Doctors often complain about the poor standard of hospital discharge letters, and this serves to demonstrate the importance of clarity in referral letters.

When contacting organizations such as the FHSA, providers, accountants and so on, it is good policy to find out to whom the letter should be addressed – with the correct title and department. The body of the letter should give enough information without being burdensome, providing the addressee with precise requests for the course of action envisaged.

The facility now exists for practices, hospitals, laboratories, FHSAs and health authorities to be linked via a computer providing a complex networking facility. Working with computers is discussed in Chapter 7.

Interpersonal communication

As we develop and grow, so we learn how to behave in a socially acceptable way by being sensitive to human behaviour. For example, a new manager should begin her job by observing and listening, and noting what appears to be the style of the practice. To rush straight in with new ideas and making drastic changes – however much they may be needed – would indicate a lack of social skill, and probably would be counter-productive.

We must therefore develop our skills in communicating with each other:

- avoid jargon
- ask open questions
- avoid ambiguity
- avoid interrupting
- give eye contact
- repeat information
- show interest
- observe body language.

It is worth considering how we ourselves feel if we are treated like an annoying interruption or as though we are stupid. We can get upset if people ignore us or if we are kept waiting without an explanation or apology. Nobody likes to be expected to remember complicated instructions or not to be looked at when being spoken to. We all respond more positively when people greet us or say goodbye to us with a smile.

Confidentiality

Communication has been discussed here in terms of giving and receiving information. It is essential that the practice manager, in her key role, ensures that all members of staff are instructed from the beginning with regard to the need to maintain a high degree of confidentiality. It should be an enforced rule, a good example being set by the doctors and the practice manager. Guidelines must be established so that all staff are confident about what information may be given and to whom, either on the telephone or at the reception desk – for example, if an employer enquires if an employee has been to see the doctor.

The performance review (see also page 63 'Appraisal')

The performance of the team, and therefore of the individuals, must be reviewed regularly. This involves looking at past and current performance, strengths and weaknesses and at positive action to improve performance. Also discussed can be potential and future prospects. Methods for doing this include self-appraisal, peer appraisal and staff appraisal.

It is essential that those being reviewed are fully aware of the aims and objectives of the review procedure, and that they do not relate it to performance-related pay. A questionnaire filled in by the employee before the review will be a useful aid, as this should reveal how they perceive their personal strengths and weaknesses, and what they feel could be done to help them to do their job better. She can also identify areas where she needs support or training to extend her skills.

The answers may then be compared with the manager's view and differences in perception can be explored during the interview. A positive plan for resolving problems and agreeing future action can be discussed.

Preparation for the interview

- Give the member of staff sufficient warning to allow them to prepare for the review.
- Ask them to think about their own performance.
- Study the job description and targets.
- Consult with others who might have a relevant contribution to the assessment.
- Allow adequate time.

The room should preferably be neutral territory, with no interruptions such as telephones. Have the appropriate paperwork to hand and be prepared to offer water and tissues! An informal setting is less threatening. Two chairs directly in front of each other make for a confrontational atmosphere; placing them slightly at an angle to each other will be much more helpful.

The interview

Start by establishing rapport with the individual; be aware of body language and mood – yours as well as the employee's. Be prepared to deal with conflict if it arises.

- Put the employee at ease.
- State the purpose of the interview.
- Ask 'open' questions, allowing the employee sufficient time to talk through the points raised.
- Summarize the points as they are covered.
- Summarize at the end, agreeing action.

After the interview

- Complete the appraisal form and show it to the employee.
- Allow for comment in writing.
- Take steps to implement the agreed action.
- Follow up to ensure that the action has taken place.

Communication to help employees

Counselling

Counselling is defined as 'assisting individuals towards independence or self-actualization' – the processes enabling a person to make his or her own decisions or choices. It is listening; guiding; communicating; giving information; pointing out options; observing. It is *not* doing all the talking, lecturing, dominating, giving solutions, pushing, judging or assuming.

Counselling can be used to prevent a problem or to help someone to work through a problem.

Assessment   means helping employees to find out what is going wrong and what is going right in their lives. It goes on throughout the helping process.

Focus   means helping employees to identify concerns or problems in order to explore and resolve them.

New perspectives   This refers to helping employees to view themselves and their concerns in such a way as to begin to see what they would like to do about them.

Goal setting   helps employees to set problem-managing goals.

Exploring possibilities   will help employees to see how goals may be accomplished; it also helps them to identify the resources that are available.

Opportunity choice   refers to helping employees to choose the kinds of opportunities that best fit their personality, resources and environment.

Programme implementation   refers to helping employees to implement the programme they have chosen – helping them to overcome the obstacles they encounter as they do so.

Evaluation   helps employees to monitor their participation in programmes/ training, achievement of their goals and management of their problem situations.

Barriers to communication

We have talked about communication in the positive sense but there are many barriers to effective communication. Some of these are:

- hierarchical status
- lack of sensitivity
- fatigue
- attitude
- personality
- agitation of the listener (eg parent of a sick child)
- lack of motivation
- exclusion of people outside the organization
- lack of consistency – everyone does not receive the same message
- poor recording – inaccurate information given
- lack of information (perhaps lack of training?)
- too much information
- inappropriate time, place or method of communicating
- lack of time
- misdirection of written communication
- inadequate preparation (eg for meetings)
- lack of structure.

Once you are aware of the barriers that may exist, you can look out for them and try to prevent them or at least minimize their effects.

Wider communication

Face-to-face communication with an individual is generally more effective than telephoning, which in turn may be more effective than writing. The same applies when communicating with a group of people. Much of the practice manager's time is spent with groups or teams, whether in a formal or an information setting.

The point about working in groups is that the task will be completed better than by an individual working alone. General practice is an organization that functions efficiently only through team effort. The skill of managing a team lies in making sure that the various parts form a complete whole. A truly effective group is frequently one that attends regular formal meetings where the team objectives are clearly established and a jointly recognized level of communication is agreed in order to achieve cohesion. Setting up successful meetings is a highly skilled operation.

Meetings

Definition of a meeting

- A coming together of people for a common purpose.
- A hostile or competitive encounter.
- A place where things meet.

Every meeting is an opportunity to make some difference to the way things are. Things change only when the people meeting share a commitment to make it happen.

Places that we meet include:

Formally	*Informally*
board room	corridor
staff room	toilet
conference room	train
training room	kitchen
office	car journey

Casual meetings that take place in the corridor between two or more members of a practice are potentially dangerous. They lead to ill-feeling in those who are not involved, and any decision made could be useless unless the important members have been consulted.

Setting up meetings

The manager is usually responsible for convening and setting up practice meetings. These may take various forms: formal or informal, in the practice or externally, daytime, evenings or weekends, between members of the in-house teams or with other organizations (eg consultants, accountants, providers, authorities). There are also various types of meeting, as shown in Table 6.1.

Table 6.1   Types of meetings

Clinical	Policy	Training	Team management
Doctors	Practice manager	Practice manager	Practice manager
Nurses	Doctors	Doctors	Secretaries
Physiotherapists	Providers	Other agencies	Receptionists
Health visitors	Consultants		
Midwives			

Within a team the compositions of meetings can fall into several categories but some common and regular ones comprise:

1 doctors and practice manager
2 doctors and employed staff
3 practice manager and staff
4 doctors and nurses – with or without the manager
5 all groups, to include the primary health care team, accountant, solicitor, FHSA, health authority, drug companies.

Formal meetings

Although the practice manager may not act as chairman, it is as well if she can ensure that the essential tasks have been attended to. It is the chairman's responsibility to prepare for the meeting by setting an agenda and advising all expected participants of the date, time and place of the meeting.

Before calling a meeting, it is worth asking:

- why hold it?
- is there a cheaper, more efficient option?
- who needs to be there?
- when does it need to be held?
- where is it best held?
- how long does it need to last?

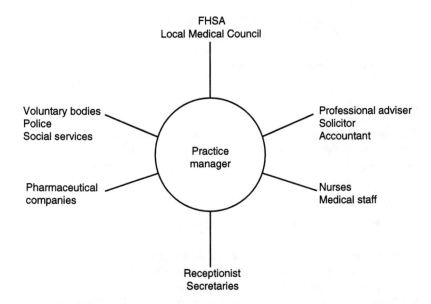

Figure 6.2:   The manager is at the centre of activities in the practice.

An ideal maximum length of time for a meeting is one to one and a half hours, as this is the maximum attention span for the majority of people.

The *main benefits* of a meeting are:

- it allows people to meet face to face
- you can see each other's reactions
- all participants learn first hand
- it allows space and pace for the information to be imparted
- it provides a wide range of experience to draw on
- it is possible to 'hear' what people are *not* saying.

All meetings need an *agenda* – there are no exceptions.

- List each item, beginning 'To . . . [*then what you want to achieve*]'
- Meetings are costly in time, so be sure to include only items that need a group decision.
- With each item, give the initials of the person responsible for bringing the topic to the meeting.
- Try to decide how long each item should take.
- Send out the agenda in good time for people to prepare for the discussion (including the chairman!).
- Supporting documents and minutes of the last meeting should be circulated with the agenda.

A *successful meeting*:

- starts and finishes on time
- ensures that all attending participate in some way
- ensures that all attending know what has been agreed
- achieves the objectives set in the (timed) agenda
- will have the minutes distributed within 24–48 hours.

Chairman

This important role should preferably be undertaken for a period of time – say 12 months or six meetings, to promote continuity. When the practice manager acts as chairman this is an ideal opportunity to develop trust and confidence with the group.

If you are in charge of the meeting:

- get to the meeting room early, having checked that it is ready
- arrange your own papers
- welcome people as they arrive, introducing visitors
- sit down before the starting time so that others follow
- check that everyone has the relevant papers
- *Start on time* (the only exception to this is when a key person is unavoidably delayed).

Chairing a meeting may come naturally to some but most people have to learn the skills required in this complex role. You must start the meeting by ensuring that everyone knows the purpose of the meeting and the items for discussion. Then you must keep a balance between controlling the meeting and the agenda, while allowing flexibility and freedom of expression. Individual differences should be respected and open discussion invited. Encourage those who indicate a desire to speak, but make sure that everyone has an opportunity to express their point of view.

The following are some suggestions for dealing with different types of people who attend meetings.

the overtalkative	break in to summarize what has been said
the wallflower	put them at their ease, and invite them to speak
the willing horse	make sure that they are going to spread the load of what they have taken on
the negative thinker	good for a balance, but build on positive points
the monkey	you cannot afford mischief makers – OUT!

Try asking more 'open' questions and fewer 'closed' ones. Open up new ideas with 'Suppose', 'Imagine' or 'What if'. Learn to listen: you have two ears and one mouth – use them in proportion. Watch what the body language is saying, and encourage others with a nod or some other sign of agreement. Learn to summarize by saying something like 'As I understand it . . .'.

It is perfectly acceptable to put your own points across but, if you do disagree, concentrate on the point not the person. It is better to agree a positive point and then disagree about something.

You must then look for areas of agreement, and reflect and summarize progress towards a decision. The five stages for reaching decisions at meetings are:

1 Introduce and define the aim
2 Examine the information
3 Generate possible solutions by encouraging discussion, and summarizing regularly
4 Make the decision (and confirm it for the minute taker and so that everyone is clear)
5 Review and revise later.

Not only must decisions be as rational as possible but they must also be accepted by the group, particularly by those who have to carry out the decisions. Otherwise, there may be a decision on paper but no subsequent action.

Minutes

It is essential that the minute taker be on time for the meeting and that the decisions taken are summarized by the chairman for accurate recording. It is a good idea to confirm in the minutes who is responsible for any *action* to be taken, and by when. It might help to have an 'action' column on the right-hand side of the minutes.

It is not necessary to record in detail the discussion of each topic but it might be helpful to record pros and cons voiced regarding a contentious item.

Informal meetings

There may be occasions when less formal meetings are appropriate; for example, when there are vague problems or specific problems between individuals. These meetings may take the form of 'buzz groups'.

7 Computers and General Practice

Why computerize?

MANY practices realize that, with the greater and ever-changing and challenging demands of the GP contract, it has become well nigh impossible to operate without a computer-based management system. The safe storage of data, its easy access, combined with the analytical capability of a reliable machine give the primary health care team the scope for effectiveness and efficiency in administration, which facilitates excellence in patient care!

Experience suggests that practices choosing to computerize or upgrade to one of the major systems for fund-holding purposes should certainly give time for the practice to adapt and develop before entering their preparatory year.

Choosing a good software system

Although much depends on the size of the practice, there will be common requirements when it comes to choosing a good software package. Some companies will sell their software separately and this may be run on a variety of machines. However, practices should be cautious about this type of agreement, as arranging support may be difficult and costly in time when breakdowns occur. Experience has proved that, as the organization increases in size and develops its use of the computer, the minimum down-time is a must. In fact, it becomes wholly unacceptable for the main processor or even a single terminal or printer to be out of action at all.

The importance of installing the most suitable software package into a practice cannot be emphasized too strongly, not least because of the initial capital outlay. Moreover, if a practice decides to convert its data to run on another system, there will be a further cost implication in that precious time will have to be given to the task, there will be unavoidable disruption, data will almost certainly be lost and a re-training programme will have to be organized.

Practices must accept that gathering, sifting and presenting information on any new idea takes time, but if this time is given freely, mistakes should not occur and the most suitable system for the practice will be chosen. Apart from the vast amount of sales literature available, unbiased advice and information may be obtained from the Royal College of General Practitioners, the Local Medical Committee and the Regional Adviser. Practices should also enlist the help of the Computer Facilitator at their FHSA, who will tell them about existing computer sites in their locality, together with the names of the systems they are running.

There is no doubt that talking to the staff and doctors in other practices using the favoured systems is essential. It is necessary to be shown ease of use in a working environment, to enquire about the quality of the product and its shortcomings, and to ask about training and back-up from the company when help is needed. It is important also to know which classification of diseases is used, and how often the drug and disease dictionaries are updated. Enquire about the frequency and standard of software upgrades, and, if relevant, apply this to the fund-holding module. Lastly, look at the system manuals, and find out how 'friendly' and comprehensive the other practice finds them in solving problems or queries.

Trade exhibitions are very useful for making comparisons. Think of a series of everyday tasks carried out in the practice and ask the sales staff on different stands to display the ease with which these can be undertaken using their system. Find out about any additional packages available, and compare the costs of these and also of system upgrades and maintenance charges.

Some of the basic facilities any computer system should offer are:

- an up-to-date patient register
- user-friendly clinical note entry
- rapid access to patient data
- a time-saving repeat prescribing facility with labelling
- if a dispensing practice, the choice of a stock control package and on-line drug ordering
- patient call and recall reporting
- recognized drug and disease classification indices
- GP contract monitoring/reporting
- a word-processing package
- on-screen prompts for 'opportunistic' screening
- an annual report generator
- on-line access to other databases, hospitals
- modem link for upload and download of data to the FHSA.

Additional facilities that should be available are:

- fund-holding software
- accounts and spreadsheet package
- payroll package
- on-screen protocols

- graphics package
- appointments module.

Introducing computerization to the practice

Although the final decision on the choice of system must be left to the partners, involving staff at the planning stage has been proved to lead to a smoother implementation programme. Doctors and practice managers who respect the feelings of their staff, realize that computerization must vastly change their jobs, and anxieties about this can easily build up and lead to a reduction in performance.

One of the best ways of introducing the concept of computerization to the staff is in open discussion with all the partners and the practice manager. It is probable that the staff will use the system more than the doctors, especially for administration, and will look at things from a different perspective.

It is vital to define and prioritize objectives for short- and long-term implementation by the identification of the main tasks requiring immediate computerization. It is essential to try to encourage everyone to take part, certainly to motivate the staff. The partners should show a combined confident front, while trying to show an understanding for the forthcoming changes. The next step is to check your specification against the features of the systems available on the market.

Using a short-list, it is necessary to arrange in-house demonstrations, making sure that the companies involved understand your need of a single- or multi-user system. Be warned that, in the current environment, a single-user system is proving inadequate; if you decide to start in this way, be sure to ascertain whether it is possible to upgrade to multi-terminal or a networked installation, at a reasonable cost.

Plan the demonstrations so that everyone can be there to try the system. Be sure to get as many views as possible afterwards and try to cover some of the same issues each time.

Here are a number of useful questions to supplement those from the practice.

- How committed are the company to GP computing?
- Can the software handle an FHSA download of the practice age/sex register; if further information, such as smear recalls or FP1001 claim status, is made available on tape or disc from the FHSA, can this data be loaded directly, on system commissioning?
- How long has the company been around, what is their development programme and how sound is their financial backing?

- What is the company's response time for help-line calls and how long is the delay for a hardware call-out? (Hardware call-out should be eight working hours or less)
- How many people in the company are involved in support?
- What time guarantees do they give in having a practice up and running after a problem, either hardware or software?
- How much training is offered free?
- How much does extra and advanced personnel training cost?
- Does the company support user-groups, and are there any locally based?

Practices should be wary of representatives who come along with rigidly rehearsed demonstrations and those who use an unacceptable amount of trade jargon. The database on the portable computer being used in these situations is often not large, which may give the impression that the speed of screen responses generally is much faster than it truly is.

Each practice will have its own requirements, because of the differences from one another in organizational terms. When it comes to making that final choice, though, cost will figure dramatically both in capital outlay and ongoing maintenance, so it is necessary to get a comparable written quotation from each of the preferred suppliers.

Preparing for the system

Once the practice has decided which computer system it is going to purchase, there must then be an organized and effective period of preparation.

If the system is to be single-user, it is essential to try to install it somewhere quiet but accessible. However, if the installation is to be multi-user, there is much to do to plan the siting of the main processor and the various terminals and printers. The same applies if the system is to contain a number of networked processors.

Involve in the planning process those of the team who are to be using the workstations, and liaise with your supplier for advice and assistance. It is no good installing a noisy printer next to the main incoming telephone extension or at the side of a busy reception desk, even if it is useful and convenient for printing repeat prescriptions!

The following points may be helpful in planning the installation.

- Decide on the positions of terminals and printers, and make sure that there are adequate power points.
- Arrange a timetable for the engineers to install cable in the surgery, and make sure that the wiring is going to be as unobtrusive as is possible.

- Where consulting room terminals are concerned, try to ensure that the terminal is strategically placed and does not intrude into the consultation setting more than it has to.
- Order all necessary stationery supplies, including FP10 Comps, floppy discs or tapes for an adequate back-up routine and also printer cartridges and ribbons.
- As some practice registers are said to be 10–20% inaccurate, it may be necessary for a validation exercise to be undertaken, using a print-out, from the FHSA. Once the practice is sure that the information is correct, and the FHSA has made any necessary changes to its database, a download of patient data may be requested.
- Health and safety standards must be met, so consider this when purchasing equipment and furniture for workstations.
- Discuss health and safety standards with all staff who will be spending much (or all) of their time entering data, and explain the need for regular breaks.
- With the software supplier, draw up a list of security passwords to allow different levels of access to the computer. Explain to all accessing personnel that they will be expected to memorize their password and keep it confidential. Do not forget to stress the importance of compliance with the regulations surrounding data protection, together with the legal implications if rules are flouted.

Personnel training

It is a recognized fact that no computer system, however simple or sophisticated to operate in a practice, will come anywhere near reaching its potential. However, if there exists commitment from a core group within the practice, who are prepared to train and motivate the rest, this may promote confidence for the future expansion of team skills. Indeed, when the system is commissioned, free training should be made a condition of purchasing the software package, and this must be used wisely and effectively by the core group.

Experience has shown that at least two members of the practice should be trained in the basic operation of the computer, including the technique necessary to make back-up copies of practice data files.

Teaching staff in pairs can also be beneficial in promoting confidence, as what one person will remember, the other won't and vice versa. Each of the pair will look to support the other and will be offered the same in return, particularly in the initial stages, when problems arise or new areas of the software are being explored.

A suggested plan of action

- Select key personnel to undertake any initial free training that is made available by the software company.
- Ascertain how much further training would cost and take advice from the trainer about planning for this.
- At the end of the initial in-house training day, be sure that the core team knows the routines for the start-up and shut-down of the computer and for taking back-up copies on to floppy discs or magnetic tapes.
- Make one or two people responsible for the computer and give them time to develop their skills.
- Keep a dialogue going with all members of the team and talk through plans for initial and on-going training programmes.
- If there is a lot of resistance or anxiety, consider employing someone with computer skills, perhaps on a short-term basis, to give confidence and training to in-house personnel.
- Do not leave all computer use to a small group of staff; try to encourage everyone to use the keyboard, if only for accessing basic information.
- As time goes on, and staff increase their knowledge of procedures, make sure they train others in the practice.
- Perhaps, through the password system, restrict access to more complicated data entry and retrieval to the more computer-capable on the team.
- Make someone responsible for ordering stationery supplies such as printer ribbons and cartridges, floppy discs, computerized FP10s and continuous paper.
- Set up and keep a written log for system problems, both hardware and software.
- Be patient. Although there is great pressure to work quickly in the current climate, it is estimated that it may be up to 12 months before a practice is using the system confidently and effectively.
- If the system is to be used in the consulting room, make provision for doctor training at convenient times and decide on a particular partner or partners who will join the core group.
- Be tolerant. Some members of the team will need more training than others; organize this to be done off-site if necessary and do not cram too much in at any one session.

It is important to remember that a well organized system training programme must be given top priority; as you increase personnel access to the computer, you increase the chances for inaccurate data recording. Training staff well, as your need to access, add to and update information increases, will mean the least disruption and should help to motivate the whole team.

Patient database

As systems have developed, it has become clear that a fully comprehensive database system is necessary to run practice administration efficiently and to keep accessible and meaningful medical records. Most systems seem to be divided into three main modules: the first contains patient registration data, the second clinical information and the third a drug dictionary together with prescribing data. The machine then has the facility to search these areas in order to retrieve information for a number of specified purposes and reasons such as screening, medical reports or to analyse data for audit purposes.

Patient register

If it is decided to input all the registered patients' information from the Lloyd George medical record envelopes, the practice must be prepared to give a considerable amount of time for this laborious task to be completed as accurately as possible. It should also be pointed out that the system cannot really be used at all until *all* basic details of patients are keyed in.

Provided the chosen system can accept an FHSA registration data download and a decision is made to order this (to be supplied either on floppy disc or magnetic tape), the practice can begin using the new machine on commissioning day. Most FHSAs normally charge a nominal fee for this service, but, provided the data have been checked beforehand, this will give the practice a fairly 'clean' database with which to kick off the new venture.

Whichever method is chosen, eventually the system will have its own electronic age/sex register containing the following data:

- Patient name
- Telephone number
- Registered doctor
- Patient address
- Sex of patient
- Date of registration
- Post code
- NHS number
- Family group

The system can be maintained accurately to reflect the practice list, allowing searches for individual patients by any of the above criteria or for groups of patients. In order to save paper, it is wise at the beginning to bring reports up on the screen before printing, to be sure that the correct group or cohort has been requested.

It must be decided, at the outset, whether patients' manual records that have been removed on an FP22 request are to be deleted from the computer or, if the software allows, categorized as 'moved away'. It has been proved useful to be able to view the records of patients who have left the practice; if, for instance, they are students and, therefore, are seen as temporary residents, the doctor can prescribe, if it is necessary, with more confidence.

It is essential, however, where a practice is notified directly of a patient's death, that it should not wait for the FP22. There should be a standard procedure to mark the computer record in some way that the patient is deceased, so that this record is not included in any recall reporting.

Patient medication

For team motivation, it is important to show, quite quickly, that this new tool is not just a glorified age/sex register. Therefore, as computers are really useful for repetitive tasks, organizing the task of loading repeat prescription details should be made a priority.

In order to keep the database accurate, and not to inconvenience the patient, it is best to write the prescription as usual, and keep a copy for checking by the doctor before the information is keyed in. It is usually necessary to specify to the computer the number of repeat prescriptions of a particular medication that will be allowed before the patient needs to attend for review. The result will mean that, for example, when six out of six prescriptions have been printed, a practice-configurable message will appear on the right-hand tear-off strip of the FP10 Comp, which will request the patient to make an appointment to be seen by the doctor before he or she is due to order a further supply. The computer will not print further prescriptions until a newly authorized number of repeats is keyed in during, or following, the review consultation.

Features of the system that are useful in relation to storing medication details are:

- printing of dispensing labels
- regular drug dictionary updates
- record of batch numbers
- check for contraindications and interactions
- check for patient compliance
- check for patient over-ordering of repeat medication
- GP monitoring system for repeat prescriptions
- stock control system
- easy identification of a patient or a group of patients on a specific therapy.

By loading this information on a phased basis, both staff and doctors will gain valuable experience fairly painlessly. The task should be completed within weeks, so that all concerned may quite rapidly be released from the laborious, repetitive job of writing repeat prescriptions, and experience the benefit of the production of accurate and legible FP10s.

With the imposition of budget limitations and cost monitoring analysis, some systems will help in assessing the current status of indicative drug budgets, through the prescribing module. However, as the calculations are based on issued prescriptions and a considerable number of patients do not get them filled, it seems difficult as yet to use anything but the Prescribing Analysis and Cost (PACT) figures for realistic monitoring.

Clinical information

One of the most effective ways to add relevant clinical information is through the use of consulting and treatment room terminals. Following training, many doctors and nurses, in some of their first 'live' patient consultations, begin by keying-in to the computer a simply coded firm or tentative diagnosis. Where applicable, this is followed by entering information related to a single prescription or perhaps is connected by authorized repeat medication. Many doctors' room terminals have quiet-running printers connected to them, so, if there is a need to prescribe, the patient leaves the consultation with a legible and accurate freshly printed and signed prescription.

If, however, the surgery has a dispensary, the system may be set up to generate a printed medicine label and, this, along with the prescription, is printed remotely. Then the dispenser, already alerted to prepare the medication as printed out, will hand the medication to the patient without undue delay, before he or she leaves the surgery.

The 'free text' facility, which is offered in many clinical information modules, will be used more widely in practices as system operators become more proficient. Some clinical staff have long felt the need for a graphics facility in this area, but we are only just seeing signs of this development being offered as part of a clinical database. There seems to be no doubt that it takes confidence and competence to move completely from manual to computer medical record-keeping but, for meaningful retrieval for audit purposes, annual reporting and financial monitoring, this is already becoming the norm in some practices.

To avoid working from the Lloyd George medical record envelopes, which can be very clumsy and time consuming to use, a practice may be running a manual currently maintained morbidity or health risk index. Computerizing easily accessed information that was previously stored in a register or card-index format, allows for easier updating, checking, monitoring and reporting, which should relate directly to improved patient care.

With the Health Promotion Banding Structure, combined with the emphasis on asthma and diabetes in disease monitoring, patients need to be identified quickly, tracked more carefully and the results of improvements in care validated more thoroughly.

Call and recall systems

Some computer systems are able to handle FHSA downloaded data on smear and FP1001 status; if this is not possible, obtain a print-out, showing relevant personal details and recall date or due date for renewal of claim. Carrying out each of these kinds of isolated loading exercises not only provides good practice in using the system but also highlights the need for accuracy. Indeed, it is sensible to organize a validation check, perhaps by viewing a number of random entries, to make sure that the data have been transcribed correctly.

Even if a practice can obtain hard copies of information, as has been suggested, it may decide to enter details on cytology and paediatric vaccination status from existing manual records and then go through some sort of validation process. Certainly, with income target setting in these areas, it is advisable to keep staff informed of the harsh reality of the possibility of falling below target levels and incurring practice income penalties.

Computerized call and recall systems can be made to work really well if staff are committed to a standardized maintenance process. The following points may serve to operate a watertight and effective, call and recall system for cytology.

- Stress the importance of accurate data entry.
- Train at least two members of staff and make them responsible for operating the complete task.
- Make sure the entry contains
  - date of last test
  - result of last test
  - appropriate recall date
  - who performed the test.
- Design a new patient questionnaire for females joining the practice, asking for the above information; when complete medical records arrive, edit the computer record for accuracy.
- Monitor numbers of patients being called, to establish availability of nurse time.
- Update information following hysterectomy or on patient refusal of a test.
- Code entry to show that the patient's GP confirms that patient is 'not sexually active'.
- Construct a list of clinical codes for data entry.
- Establish a policy on the number of recall reminders to be sent or the number of telephone calls that will be made by, preferably, the practice nurse.
- Design appropriate letters noting that second and third reminders, if required, need to be firmer in their request for attendance.
- Experience suggests that, for a greater response, all letters are signed by the patient's GP.

Millbrook End Surgery
Caresborough
Milltown ME56 9FG

Telephone 0899 567890
Extension : F5

Thank you for attending for a smear test. It is advisable that you contact us

for the result . . . . weeks from today.

Will you please telephone our Secretary between 2pm and 5pm Tuesday to
Friday on the above number or call at our reception desk between these times.

Figure 7.1: Example of a hand-out to be given to a patient who has attended for a test.

- Give the patient a hand-out such as is shown in Figure 7.1, so that she knows whom to contact, and at a time when the surgery is quieter and has the result readily available on screen.
- Enter that the patient has attended, that a test result is awaited and alter recall date to tie up with the laboratory response time.
- Record the laboratory findings without delay, and endorse the new entry with the correct recall date. Remove the entry showing test result awaited.
- Bring any problem test results to the attention of the doctor, in order that appropriate action may be taken.
- On a regular cycle, it is necessary to run a report for any test results that are overdue from the laboratory, as a safety net.

Each call and recall system may be run on the same principle, whether it be for child immunizations, renewal of contraceptive services or any other item of service:

- complete a clinical or administrative procedure
- enter this by agreed code into the computer
- endorse the entry with the appropriate date for next contact
- update, as necessary, patients joining or leaving the practice
- run weekly or monthly reports for calls and recalls due
- call patients or review them 'opportunistically' with system prompts.

Standardization of entries

As we have seen already, there are various ways that a practice may begin to build the information stored on its database.

One of the joys of storing administrative, clinical and encounter information on a practice computer is that this record will always be accessible, and not lost in mis-filing or end up in the renowned boot of a doctor's car!

However, there must be a disciplined approach as to where specified information should appear in the patient record and, perhaps, by using agreed protocols, which codes are the most acceptable and useful, for recording particular morbidity data.

The 'garbage in–garbage out (GI–GO) statement may never be more true than when poor system housekeeping is in place. Enthusiasm can be difficult to harness, but channel it carefully and constructively, with training and a controlled approach, and the whole team will see and reap the benefits. However, a computer system added to a practice that is normally managed chaotically will cause further frustration and demotivation.

Classic examples of poor discipline are the codes used for chest problems, which may be wide ranging. When the partners request a report to be generated showing those patients suffering from asthma or chest-related conditions, it is difficult to be confident in the results. How can a practice hope to plan the care of this group of patients if it does not know how many there are, how often they attend or whether they have been seen recently?

Begin by enforcing the statement that an inaccurate and untidy database is useless. Computers cost a great deal, but this is the tip of the iceberg when we consider the time spent entering information. If that information cannot be accessed or retrieved in a reliable and useful format, it would be as well not to bother at all.

Some points to ponder are as follows:

- Consider the database to be 'clean' at commissioning of the system.
- Do everything you can to preserve the cleanliness of your data.
- Never forget the GI–GO factor.
- Set up random validation and accuracy-check processes.
- Tackle computerization in your surgery like the eating of an elephant: take it *a bite at a time.*
- In the early stages, restrict data entry to a small number of people and give access-only passwords to the others.
- Encourage clinical staff to work on developing data entry protocols, and to plan where this information will be held in the patient records.
- Continually enforce the value of getting it right and keeping it that way.

Some medical systems now offer software that allows the practice to programme in its own defined protocols for both clinical and administrative data entry. This method will enable greater standardization of the use of codes, leading to much more accurate reporting. Currently, it is still quite complex to find and enter all the variable codes but this is sure to become simpler as systems develop further.

General practitioners are being told to record such details of a patient as body mass index (BMI). Some systems allow particular codes to be entered for height and weight and will work out the BMI automatically from these readings. A prompt can then be made to appear on the screen for the doctor or nurse to counsel the patient regarding diet and losing or gaining weight as necessary. The same system may be used to collect health check data, and prompts may be set up for each question regarding smoking and alcohol status and for recording family history and risk factors.

New ideas tend to generate more work. Information technology is being developed to try to ease the administrative burden on practices but everyone on the team needs to co-operate.

Appointment systems and address book

Appointment diary

Commerce has been operating computerized appointment diaries for many years, but it is only recently that medical practices have begun to move to this method of booking patients' appointments.

The greatest advantage of using an automated system is that most seem to offer the booking facility to receptionists who greet patients at the appointment desk and on the telephone, and to doctors or nurses from their consulting rooms.

As each patients arrives, the listed appointment is endorsed accordingly; the same happens if a patient cancels during a clinic or a surgery session. If another patient is slotted into a cancelled slot, or there were gaps available after the start of the session, the list is edited and the doctor or nurse viewing the updated screen should have no problem in calling the correct patient.

An extra free text field is available on some systems so that, if patients tell the receptionist why they wish to be seen, this can be added to the screen.

Where there are land-lines between branch and main surgeries, the system becomes invaluable. For example, a doctor working at the branch may wish to see the patient at the main surgery on another day, and may book the appointment remotely, an impressive administrative capability.

The system must be able to cope with being programmed for doctors' half-days, bank holidays and week-ends. Because the data are reliable and accurate, a picture of throughputs of workload can be easily drawn and used as a planning tool when reviewing the overall structure or individual clinics or sessions.

A built-in printing facility, to offer hard copies of the session lists, is usually available for those sites that do not have terminals in every consulting and treatment room.

The biggest single problem with using a computerized appointment diary is the threat of a system breakdown or power cut, as this will directly affect the patient being offered a new or a change of appointment upon request. Practices should look to their supplier for advice about using a continuous power supply unit which, in the event of a power cut, gives time for the session lists to be printed before the computer is temporarily closed down.

Address book

A very useful facility available on most of the leading medical systems is an address book. If this is fully integrated, it provides an easily accessible record of an individual patient's previous place of residence when a change of address is notified and the registration record has been edited and, therefore, shows on screen only the new address. Another helpful feature here is that it is possible to store the name of a next of kin connected to a patient's name, and this may be easily retrieved if there is a problem or an emergency occurs.

A practice nurse, secretary or receptionist is often asked for a contact address or telephone number for national or local self-help groups, covering many aspects of health and social care, and this is where an address book is invaluable. Patients are quite impressed when practice staff have this kind of information at their fingertips.

This module gives space to record staff and doctors' home addresses. It may also be used to list addresses and telephone numbers for contacting all other members of the primary health care team, including social workers.

Effective use of the address book facility will put an end to time-wasting scanning of telephone directories, files or correspondence for commonly used contact addresses.

Word processing

For a practice to get the very best out of any word-processing package, there must be assessment of the expected quality of the finished document and an on-going training programme. Hardware costs continue to be more competitive, so a sophisticated laser printer, capable of producing an extremely high standard of printed document, connected to a stand-alone IBM-compatible processor (ideally a 386 or 486 machine) is well within the reach of even some of the smaller practices. The addition of a mouse, complete with mat, will allow speed of access to drop-down 'menus'.

Many local evening classes and technical colleges run training courses in the standard packages. Alternatively, practices can contact commercial organizations that offer personalized sessions on- or off-site using the package installed on the practice computer. As many of the official manuals are quite unhelpful, it is as well to look around for a simplified version.

Surgeries can now design their own headed paper to be produced in-house, thus avoiding expensive printing bills for letterheads, compliments and appointment slips. Patient advice sheets, news-sheets and even practice leaflets may be regularly updated and printed at a fraction of their original cost.

There are a wide variety of word-processing packages, commercially available, offering many of the following advantages over using a standard typewriter:

- printing of a pre-configured and stored practice letter
- effortless text editing
- enhancement of text for adding more interest to documents such as the annual report
- endless flexibility in setting out documentation
- automatic numbering of pages
- storage for copies of letters, avoiding excessive waste of paper
- spell-checking facility
- integrated thesaurus to allow the broader use of vocabulary
- the compilation and storage of frequently used and standardized letters for editing and 'mail-merging'
- any number of copies of a top-copy standard
- the capacity to cut text from a file and either paste it somewhere else in the same document or enter it directly into a separate letter or report
- graphics capability.

Integrated word-processing software

Many of the major medical system suppliers provide a word-processing module as part of the standard package, even though it may not always be fully integrated. The use of a word processor may not be a practice priority in choosing a main system but should be considered. If there is a possibility of future development for producing standard call and recall letters and patient referral correspondence, which will allow the use of a mail-merge facility from the medical database, incorporating word processing in the system will avoid the time-wasting double-entry of data. The packages offered in this way are often more basic and do not contain the same graphics sophistication as those operating in a 'Windows' environment which seem to allow the user to complete quite sophisticated tasks quite easily.

Many systems use the integrated word processor to:

- generate patient medical records in text form for easy editing before making hard copies

- produce practice personalized standard letters
- mail-merge personalized standard letters to the report generator
- produce simple graphs and histograms.

Financial packages

There are a host of financial packages, some written especially with general practice in mind and some that are commercially standard. The term 'financial package' is used to cover accounts and spreadsheet software and, if used well to prepare the practice accounts, can not only save on accountants' costs but also give the practice up-to-the-minute meaningful management information at its fingertips for both short- and long-term planning.

Most suitable packages are run on an MS-DOS operating system but many medical systems run on other types such as BOS, Xenix or MUMPS, which are incompatible. Nevertheless, the practice may be able to ascertain from their main computer supplier whether their hard disk could be partitioned to run two operating systems, or it may choose to purchase a stand-alone IBM-compatible processor of 386 or 486 power, as was mentioned in the section 'Word processing'. The latter suggestion seems to be the way forward for many practices in developing their use of accounts, spreadsheet and payroll on one machine. This can, in turn, be networked to another machine running word processing. In order to keep costs down, it is possible to connect one printer to this network, which allows printing access from all loaded packages.

As internal security is paramount with such sensitive data, practices must ensure that they have the facility to implement a strict user password system.

Accounts packages

It is clear that many accounts packages can do much more for the practice than just keep an electronic record of book-keeping transactions. The data may be used for management analysis in varying formats:

- graphical
- individual doctor
- item of service claims
- time period reports
- target payments
- claims by value and number
- clinic or minor surgery claims
- superannuation statements

Practices may choose just to run a simple *cash book*, which records income and expenditure. This does not allow the tracking of assets and liabilities and so will not produce a balance sheet to go forward for the presentation of final accounts.

If the practice chooses a full *nominal ledger* package, this has the capacity to produce full and final accounts, which minimizes the work undertaken by the practice accountant at the end of the financial year.

The cash book is there to control such areas as petty cash, multiple bank accounts, standing order and direct debit payments. Regular bank reconciliation, essential to any business, is made simple and most packages provide an audit trail facility. There may be provision here for the partners' capital accounts.

Some of the features of a comprehensive ledger system are:

- cash book
- purchase ledger
- partners' ledger
- nominal ledger
- report generator
- FHSA ledger

For a practice to be able to maintain an effective claiming procedure, it is necessary also for expenditure on rent and rates and staff salaries to be easily defined. A practice also needs to validate payment of all FHSA claims, and computerizing the accounts can make this task much more effective and less time-consuming.

Payroll

Up to a few years ago, it was an accepted fact that you needed many more employees than the average practice to justify the purchase of a payroll package. However, as suitable software is now readily available at prices that will not break the bank, many practices are choosing this method for the calculation of staff salaries, budget reconciliation and FHSA returns.

Some salary packages come as a separate module integrated into an accounts package; others may be bought in addition. Payroll data that imports directly into the accounts not only saves time but also leads to greater accuracy without the need of double-entry, which can cause error.

As moving to a completely new electronic system takes confidence, many practices choose to calculate one month's salaries manually and also run them off the computer. It should be possible to view the payslips before printing to allow a validation check, giving the operator the chance to correct any differences or errors in operation before abandoning what is a very repetitive and time-consuming task.

Features to look for when choosing a suitable package are:

- cash payments
- credit transfers
- overtime payments
- weekly and monthly payments

- SSP and SMP
- P60, P35 and P45

- trainee and associate GP salaries
- FHSA variable rate returns

The rates for PAYE and National Insurance change from year to year, so it is necessary to check the charges made to be supplied with these regular updates.

Spreadsheets

A spreadsheet package is one that can simplify the handling of figures when undertaking complicated calculations. Practical everyday use of a spreadsheet gives a practice the capacity to examine the current status and to project the effect of maintaining this or of introducing variance.

Modern packages offer a graphics facility and space to add text, making report compilation easier and more interesting. Cash flow forecasts, normally presented in tabular form, will be easily produced. Provided all the figures are accurate and placed in the correct columns, a clear picture can easily be presented.

Spreadsheets can have a very practical application. They may be used to demonstrate the effect of a rise in staff salary costs, or changes in expected income with the arrangements regarding health promotion payments.

The most common use of spreadsheets in general practice seems to be in analysing the data in the practice accounts. A spreadsheet can take the stored figures relating to income and expenditure and make the accountant's job easier by tracking what money is being generated and where it is being spent. Manually, a practice may break down its income and expenditure into a few named columns but, by using a spreadsheet with imported data from an accounts package, the analysis will be in a much clearer and presentable form. The value of graphics to present sources of income and expenditure to the partners cannot be overestimated and gives rise to a more professional approach to business planning.

Health and safety standards

Since the beginning of 1993, any new workstations bought for use in a commercial environment in the UK must conform to an EC Directive. These guidelines have been introduced to protect personnel who use a visual display unit (VDU) from health risk involving work-related upper limb disorder (WRULD), repetitive strain injury (RSI), visual fatigue and stress. For existing workstations, employers have until 31 December 1996 to bring them into line with these standards.

It is necessary to assess who in the practice is covered by the Directive but it suggests that it is anyone who uses a VDU for an hour or more at a time. This means at least all secretaries using word processors and data-entry operators, particularly if in a fund-holding practice; at most it could include the doctors, nurses and receptionists, if the practice is using the system throughout.

Individuals must be assessed and a written record of this kept on file. Employees are entitled to a copy of their risk assessment and any steps the practice is taking to minimize any future effects.

Guidelines

The term 'workstation' refers to both the VDU and the desk area used in relation to it.

Screens   These need to be readable, adjustable and glare-free

Keyboards   These must be comfortable to use, adjustable, and the keytops must be legible

Desk surfaces   Give space to work, allow flexible arrangements and supply text-holders if appropriate

Chairs   Make these adjustable and supporting, and provide foot rests

Floor area   Be sure to provide a reasonable amount of leg room

Lighting   Prevent glare and reflection, and provide adequate contrast and comfortable light

Noise   Keep distracting noise to a minimum

Humidity   Avoid excessive heat, and provide adequate humidity and ventilation

Software   Make sure that this is appropriate for the task and that staff are trained adequately to be capable users

Staff working with VDUs now have the right to an eye test at the employer's expense, though they may choose not to take this up.

In order to alleviate boredom and eye strain and to keep stress levels down, it is necessary to vary the workload and routine to include rest breaks from using a VDU. It is suggested that a five-minute break in every hour is acceptable, and that a task away from the desk area is preferable.

Practices can obtain information and help from the Health and Safety Executive, who have a number of booklets available. It is also possible to take advice from your computer supplier and office equipment specialist when purchasing or renewing furniture or computers.

Data Protection Act

It must be stressed that every practice using a computer that holds personal information is breaking the law if it is not registered, under the Data Protection Act, with the Data Protection Registrar.

The Act is quite complex and a series of explanatory booklets have been produced as guidance. They can be obtained from the Data Protection Registry Office. The forms for registration are quite formidable to complete, so it is worth obtaining a copy of the GMSC's comprehensive guide before attempting the task.

A registration fee is payable, and it is compulsory for a practice to renew registration every three years. If a practice sells data to a third party, it must inform patients; otherwise the information may be deemed to have been obtained unfairly.

Further guidelines as to GP responsibilities in relation to the Act are available from the GMSC. They include:

- positioning of terminals so that they are turned away from casual on-lookers
- making sure that staff understand that idle screens should be logged off or blanked out
- regularly changing passwords, making sure that the correct access levels are issued
- disabling of passwords of ex-employees without delay
- never allowing complacency regarding back-up procedures
- fitting of lockable devices, to secure computers to desks
- making use of the locks on personal computer system boxes
- shredding all unwanted computer print-outs.

It is advisable to take general security advice from your computer supplier, and also to look into insuring your data in case there is permanent damage to hardware or software, involving high costs of re-inputting data.

Back-up procedure

Whether a practice decides to use floppy disks or magnetic tapes, it is necessary to complete a back-up of practice data on a daily basis. In order to prevent damage to this recorded data, the chosen back-up media should not be put next to equipment that contains magnetism or a high electrical charge (eg portable telephones) and should certainly not be taken in lifts.

The back-up disks or tapes should be stored either off the premises or in a fireproof safe or box.

Your computer supplier will, every three to six months, verify your tapes or disks, for it is not until you have had a problem and need to re-load data that you will know whether the data recorded is corrupted in any way. It is, of course, necessary for a practice to have a signed confidentiality statement included in the company maintenance agreement.

The 'grandfather–father–son' back-up concept is an accepted commercial routine:

Day 1	→	Tape 1	or	Set of daily disks labelled Monday
Day 2	→	Tape 2	or	Set of daily disks labelled Tuesday
Day 3	→	Tape 3	or	Set of daily disks labelled Wednesday
Day 4	→	Tape 1	or	Set of daily disks labelled Thursday
Day 5	→	Tape 2	or	Set of weekly disks labelled Week one

and so on.

As the example shows, there are three tape back-ups in circulation and, because of the speed of a tape streamer unit, these will probably contain a full data copy.

Because the process with floppy disks is much slower, it is possible to take a daily copy of practice data and only once a week take a full data copy. Daily disks can be overcopied, once a weekly copy of this information has been successfully taken. However, there must be three sets of disks for weekly back-ups, labelled Week one, Week two and Week three. It is essential to make sure that all back-up media is correctly labelled with date and time, and used sequentially.

Collecting data for audit

The whole concept of audit is raised when someone asks what is actually happening. Without facts, changes cannot be planned or controlled, and this is where data collection and extraction become a powerful tool.

Strict guidelines must be understood and followed by everyone involved in collecting data, and a simple system must be devised, for the strength of any such reporting is in its accuracy and therefore it is important that the GI–GO factor is appreciated by all.

To increase the chances of a satisfactory outcome of a computerized audit:

- obtain reasonable resources (eg staff/doctor time and equipment)
- allow time to achieve accuracy
- give time for training
- involve those taking part in the planning process
- decide what is measurable
- set up a mechanism for feedback of problems
- make a group decision on the codes to be used
- set time boundaries, if appropriate
- set standards and objectives, however simple
- encourage and motivate
- arrange for a validation exercise
- set up a forum to evaluate findings
- assess need for change.

Some of the main medical systems come with practice-configurable protocol screens, which may be set up for medical audit purposes as well as for administrative reasons. These screens give greater accuracy with input of data because the choice of codes offered to the operator are pre-specified and may be limited.

Application for approval into the higher bands of health promotion has encouraged many practices to collect data in this way. This means that doctors and nurses are prompted by the computer to ask patients questions such as:

Have you ever smoked?	YES/NO
Do you smoke now?	YES/NO
Do you smoke (a) cigarettes, (b) a pipe, or (c) cigars?	a/b/c

Do you drink alcohol?	YES/NO
• beer/lager	YES/NO
how many units per week?	
• wine	YES/NO
how many units per week?	
• spirit	YES/NO
how many units per week?	

The answers to these and any further required/appropriate questions will place an automatic pre-defined coded entry into the patient's computer record. They can then be searched for, to meet the latest statistical requirements for the banding structure.

The resultant data, because it has been collected in this disciplined but nevertheless easy fashion, will be both accurate and meaningful. It may then be possible to look at which group of the practice population will be targeted for, perhaps, a reduction in the numbers of smokers or which group need more exercise and dietary advice. Auditing progress in these groups of patients, over a controlled period of time, can motivate doctors and nurses as they see the effect on the practice population.

Data collection exercises may be used to plan changes in many areas of the practice, from the appointments system and realistic staffing levels to the treatment of certain diseases and conditions. Audit is here to stay and computerized practices will be invaluable aids.

Developments

Links within the NHS

The government wishes to see the main elements of the National Health Service communicating by computer during the mid-nineties. This is being worked towards in many parts of the country, as practices prepare to become linked with their FHSAs. This will mean that, using a modem and a secure electronic mailbox, registration and de-registration of patients and submission of claim forms will be performed through the keyboards of computers at either end.

With the development of Trust hospitals and their need to attract business, we shall see a much wider use of a dial-in facility for remote viewing of waiting list data. More and more hospital and private laboratories are already offering an on-line fast results service, and x-ray departments are following this trend.

Modem communications

Most of the main suppliers of general practice computer systems include a modem as part of the hardware installed, and this is sure to become standard. Some of these companies also offer a communications package, free of charge, and use a telephone link into the system for both software and hardware support as part of the maintenance agreement.

Having a modem installed gives the practice an exciting dimension in the use of their computer by allowing access to exterior medical and commercial databases, remote practice terminals and 'bulletin boards'. This process is referred to as data transfer and data exchange.

Medical databases already include drug information services and travel vaccination data. There is a public-accessed service offering health promotion advice and another showing details of the effects of harmful household substances.

A subscription is required to access commercial databases such as Prestel viewdata. Likewise, if a practice or the partners wish to communicate with the bank, in order to complete transactions by modem, a charge will be levied but this may well be cost-effective.

The potential of using off-site terminals is as yet mostly unexplored in general practice perhaps because of financial constraints. A limited number of branch surgeries are now linked by telephone to the main processor; however, little use is being made of this kind of facility from the home of any of the partners or the practice manager. A sure development of remote access will be the out-of-hours doctor carrying a portable computer which will be plugged into the telephone line in a patient's home to allow full access to the patient's stored medical record.

'Bulletin boards' are still very new in general practice computing, but those already available are developing quite quickly and providing some useful tips and information. The limiting and frustrating factor of using a bulletin board is that often only one telephone line is available.

Storage of data

Data stored in general practice computer systems is still limited by the necessity to input information through a keyboard; this is an area that will receive some priority in the next few years. Graphics capability is another, as many clinicians like to indicate the site of a clinical problem by drawing in manual notes and will want the same facility in an electronically stored medical record.

Patient-held medical record

Pilot studies of data cards, the size and shape of a plastic credit card, which are able to hold up to 1200 pages of personal health information, have been underway for some time. Machines installed in health centres, out-patient departments and pharmacies can read and update the information. Confidentiality is maintained by a series of passwords. It seems that patients in Scotland may be among the first in Great Britain to test the advantages of these so-called SMART cards.

Glossary of terms

Application	The task or group of tasks for which the computer is being used
Applications packages	A set of specialized programs and associated documentation to carry out a particular application – eg payroll
Back-up	A copy of stored data, taken mainly for reasons of safety, which is stored separately from the main system
Configuration	The chosen pieces of hardware and the connections between them for a particular period of operation
CPU	Central processing unit – the principal operating part of a computer
Cursor	A symbol (often made to blink for clarity) on a display screen that indicates the active position at which the next character will be displayed
Database	A collection of interrelated data values stored in one location on the computer system
Data entry	The process by which an input device, such as a keyboard, is used to enter data into the computer system
Data transmission	The process of sending data measurements, coded characters or general information, from a sender to one or more receivers
Download	The electronic transfer of information from one database to another
Down-time	The percentage of time during which the computer system is not available for general use
Electronic mail	A communications system by which messages are sent between users using electronic communication and storage techniques
Electronic mailbox	A holding area for documents or data that have been transmitted over telephone circuits and vice versa, to allow data transmission
Floppy disk	A lightweight magnetic disk used to store information
FP10(Comp)	NHS prescription forms printed on continuous stationery, for use in a computer-driven printer
GI–GO factor	The term 'Garbage In–Garbage Out' signifies that a system working on incorrect data, or data input incorrectly, will output incorrect results

Graphics	A type of computer output which is mainly in pictorial form given via a VDU or printer
Hard copy	See print out
Hardware	The physical part of a computer, which includes devices, circuits, drives, printers and cabinets
Information retrieval	The activity of retrieving stored information from the system
Keying-in	The process of data entry, specifically using a keyboard
Land-line	A telephone link-line between pieces of hardware at different sites
Magnetic tape	A flexible tape with a magnetic coating used to store information
Modem	A device that converts a computer's digital signals into signals that can be transmitted over telephone circuits and vice versa, thus allowing data transmission
Module	A chapter or section
Mouse	A device, operated by hand, used to move a cursor around a display screen
Mouse mat	The anti-static mat which the mouse (above) rests upon
MS-DOS	Microsoft Disk Operating System, which is commonly used on IBM-compatible computers
Multi-user system	A system that allows many users to carry out operations simultaneously
Networked installation	A number of processors linked to a central file server and a storage device
Packages	A set of programs and associated documentation to carry out a particular application
Password	A means of identification often used to gain access to the system
Printout	The output from a computer-controlled printer
Processor	The computer, usually the central processor component
Single-user system	A system that permits single-user operations only – with one CPU, one VDU and some printing capability
Software	A term describing those components of a computer system that cannot be physically identified - ie the programs and documentation
Start-up and shut-down	A pre-defined group of keystrokes used to enable entry to, or exit from, the computer system
Terminal	A computer screen, or VDU with a keyboard

Upgrade	An update of the software to remove minor errors or to add new features
User-friendly	An adjective used to indicate that the system (or package, etc) has been designed with helpful features to assist inexperienced users
VDU	Visual display unit – a computer screen or monitor
'Windows'	A user-friendly package for organizing and running applications programs
Workstation	A work location that is equipped with all the facilities to perform a particular type of task (the minimum is usually a VDU and a keyboard)

8   Managing Audit

THERE have been a number of attempts to define what is meant by medical audit. In the earlier editions of this book we described it as 'looking at what you do to see if you can do it better'. This has the advantage of being both understandable and acceptable but runs the risk of over-simplifying what is a complex undertaking. The Department of Health White Paper *Working for Patients* (published in 1989) defined it as 'the systematic, critical analysis of the quality of medical care, including the procedures used for diagnosis and treatment, the use of resources, and the resulting outcome and quality of life for the patient'. That definition carries our understanding further but has a weakness in that it fails to describe the components of audit. Hughes and Humphrey (1990) listed these as:

- defining standards, criteria, targets or protocols for good practice against which performance can be compared
- systematic gathering of objective evidence about performance
- comparing results against standards and/or among peers
- identifying deficiencies and taking action to remedy them
- monitoring the effects of action on quality.

This encapsulates what is to be done but requires further discussion.

Attitudes

You should recognize at the start the medical audit is a potentially threatening activity for all who take part in it. There is an implication which you could all admit privately that what you are doing is not always the best that could be done. Whilst it is reasonable to admit this to yourselves privately, it is not so easy to admit it to others or, more alarming still, to have it pointed out by others. Yet we are all working towards the same objectives and desire to provide the best possible care for our patients. If you can somehow get rid of the attitude that it is blameworthy to identify a deficiency, you are half way to developing the sort of personal confidence and mutual respect of others that is an indispensable condition for medical audit. This change of attitude is the first important step to take. It is easier to do it within a group of equals

– peer group – who work together, so the doctors in a practice may find it easier to start among themselves than have other staff members involved. Similarly, a group of practice nurses may find it easier to set out on the exercise without doctors being present. As confidence in the method develops, it is possible to extend audit to others working in different practices or coming from different fields of work. It will be seen that confidentiality is an important feature of this exercise, for if you are unable to be truthful then you are unable to conduct honest audit.

There is, of course, one other attitude that is important. All those who take part must see the exercise as being important and relevant to them in their work or, at any rate, in the work of the practice as a whole. They should understand that audit is a very powerful educational tool and, if carried out properly, one of the most important agencies for change that exists. For this reason the choice of audit topic is important and should be the choice of all.

Resources

The most precious resource you have is time. This has become even more obvious recently when a wide range of new activities have been thrust upon general practice. When you are busy, it may seem too much to ask for an extra hour or two each week for medical audit; yet if you do not do it, the quality of work may deteriorate, dangerous mistakes may occur and you may become even more busy for audit may reveal ways of saving time or using time more effectively. It is therefore a priority activity.

The second resource you need to access to good data. Here another important principle operates: the data used for audit should be based on that required for the normal clinical care of patients or the management of the practice. Examples of this include the clinical notes of patients, letters sent and received, emergency calls, appointments, PACT data and so on. It is a good general rule that if, in order to carry out an audit, you have to set up and collect entirely new data that you do not normally need or use, think again.

The words 'standards' and 'criteria' are so commonly used in any discussion of audit that they are worth spending a few minutes defining what we mean by them. Essentially, standards are the levels of performance the auditors have set themselves to achieve. They contain an element of judgement, for they are an amalgam of what is desirable and what is possible. It may be desirable for the doctor always to see the ear drum of a child with earache before diagnosing otitis media but an attempt to do that in a child in whom the drum is obscured by wax may have to be abandoned for the sake of not causing additional and, perhaps unnecessary, stress to the patient.

It is desirable that 'anyone asking for an appointment always receives one when they request one' but it is obviously impossible in the face of others seeking similar appointments at the same time and the limited resources available. The standard therefore requires qualification and it needs to be made explicit. For example, it may need to be qualified by saying that the appointment will be with 'a' doctor but not necessarily 'the' doctor of the patient's choice, and it may be made explicit by adding the words 'within 24 hours if not urgent'. Here we move into the realm of something that can be measured and this is termed a 'criterion'. There may be several criteria attached to a standard but as soon as even one criterion has been listed it becomes possible to measure performance. The ability to measure performance is very important to audit. Thus in this example it would be possible to see how many patients actually received an appointment within 24 hours of asking and then to continue with the various intellectual steps of the audit and analysis.

There is, however, a danger lurking within this concept. Not everything can be measured. Certainly not everything that is desirable in patient care can be measured. Furthermore, some of the most important elements of good quality patient care cannot be measured or can be measured only with the greatest difficulty and it is important not to let this produce a skewed view of the real, but limited, value of audit. Some of the elements we are talking about are such things as the quality of communications, attitudes such as courtesy and consideration. However, even these are capable of rigorous examination and you will be familiar with the discussion that takes place, often in an informal setting over coffee, in which the problems faced by a single doctor in the care of a patient are raised. The issues raised may be of a patient who fails to respond to treatment or advice, or angry relatives of a patient who died, and the doctor or nurse gets support, alternative suggestions or new perspectives from the group. 'Critical event audit' disciplines this informal activity and takes it further, for it asks not only what might be done better in relation to this case but also what lessons might be learnt from this case that are of general application. It tries to develop a standard of care from the particular against which the care of the many can be measured.

For example, a young woman in the practice who is under treatment for depression commits suicide. You might enquire what clues, if any, existed for this behaviour and how they could have been identified. You might ask what preventive measures exist, what other services are used and what are their deficiencies. You might in fact learn from this single case a pattern of activity that is better than you had before. From this you can begin to create a standard of care that you can test on other cases. It might contain a number of criteria, or factors that produce a more accurate definition of what is meant by 'depressed', what you should record, what you should do for continuity of care, how you should communicate, what should be described and how, and so on. This type of audit has the attraction that you do not need large numbers of cases before you can do it better! It also emphasizes the fact that such standards are not unchangeable. They are not written on tablets of stone. As another such audit is done, your standards may change for new drugs or new patterns of care may come along. Audit is essentially a dynamic process and should never be static.

Whilst you should not decry the value of this sort of audit – and carried out in a rigorous way it can produce effective change – most of the time when you think of medical audit you think of the sort of data described in Chapter 7. The fact that all participants in audit must feel committed to the importance and relevance of the audit has already been mentioned. This is particularly important in this form of audit when the data collected are the result of others' work. An example of this might be a decision to audit some aspects of the care of asthma.

An audit in asthma care

To create an opportunity for teamwork and address the practice's need to formulate an asthma protocol as a development in chronic disease management, a doctor, a practice nurse, a district nurse and a medical records staff member adopted the task as a project. Together they planned their approach; in the absence of a practice manager at this time, the GP undertook the role of negotiation and delegation within the team.

1 They agree *why* the practice wanted an asthma protocol:
   • asthma is common
   • effective treatment is available
   • asthma is currently managed in a haphazard way
   • asthma is a significant cause of mainly preventable morbidity and mortality.
2 The team outlines their *aims* for the care of asthmatic patients:
   • how to recognize asthma in patients
   • treatment to maximize airways function
   • minimal interference with normal lifestyle
   • reduction in morbidity and mortality
   • increasing understanding of asthma in patients and the primary health care team
   • improvement in records of patient care
   • maintenance of knowledge base – keep up to date.

To assess what information was accessible, it was necessary to perform an initial audit to provide the baseline data for later comparison. Here the team apportioned responsibility according to clinical or administrative skills. The group decided on the baseline data required:

- to identify patients and provide a register for the clinic
- to provide a baseline for future audit
- to classify patients into degree of severity in order to determine frequency of clinic attendance.

In 1987 the number of asthma patients was shown to be 2.9% of the practice population. In 1990, the figures were higher, at 5.5%. Subsequently the initial audit was carried out.

Medical records staff organized a print-out of all asthma patients giving name, address and date of birth. Asthmatic patients were identified by staff:

- from the age/sex register with associated disease diagnostic index
- from diagnosis on computer
- by searching for asthma medication.

The total number of asthmatics identified in this way was 1484 (approx. 10% of the practice population). Therefore approximately 10% of the practice population had some asthma-linked entry on their computer records.

All these patients were classified by the clinical team into severity:

mild	requiring intermittent therapy	66%
moderate	requiring regular treatment plus/minus nebulization	24%
severe	prescribed steroids/hospital admission within the past year	10%

Of the 1484 identified, a 10% sample was audited by accessing the manual patient records. Results over the course of one year (1990) were:

42% had been seen with respect to their asthma
20% had a peak expiratory flow rate (PEFR) recorded
7.5% had had an emergency appointment
5.5% had had a home visit
3.5% had had nebulization
1.4% were admitted to hospital

Total number of out-of-hours visits = 27 (from the Visits book)
Total number of admissions = 11
Total number of deaths = 0

On the basis of these results, the pros and cons for clinic-based care versus opportunistic screening were listed, and the decision was made to establish a rolling asthma clinic. Questions raised concerned who would run the clinic, when would the clinic be held, how long would the consultation be and how would records be kept.

Who?

The clinics were to be run mainly by one practice nurse and one district nurse, both participating in the project and each of whom had a special interest in asthma, having attended the Stratford Training Course on Asthma. Two doctors would provide medical back-up as required. Medical records staff would provide administrative support.

Times?

To provide flexibility and convenience for patients, who would be managed according to the protocol, the clinic would be run as a 'rolling' session (as approved for the diabetic and hypertension clinics). The nurses agreed on the desirable length of consultations and frequency of attendance:

- 30 minutes for initial appointment
- 15 minutes for follow-up appointments.

Records?

- Stratford yellow cards – flow sheets prompting entry of clinical data
- asthma clinic register – for ease of recall
- consistent computer record entries to facilitate searches in future audit
- after the session, patient records were sent to the medical records office for verification of data and accurate claims procedure for health promotion funding.

Which patients?

If all known asthmatics were seen once a year, 28 additional appointments would be required per week. If patients with moderate/severe asthma were seen twice a year and the remainder once a year, 38 additional appointments per week would be needed. Therefore, initially, it was necessary to prioritize:

- all new diagnoses of asthma
- all new registrations of known asthmatics (NB combine with new patient check)
- all patients seen acutely for nebulizer/steroids/admission (i.e. opportunistic pick-up by GPs of patients with on-going problems)
- start recall of patients in 'severe/moderate' category (this group can be identified via the computer prescriptions of Becloforte).

Having prepared the framework, the team drew up a clear protocol for the asthma clinic, shown in Box 8.1.

Box 8.1: Asthma clinic protocol

Initial appointment

- registration details
- full history
- blood pressure
- urine if on oral steroids

All appointments

- symptoms:
  - night-time waking
  - perceived limitation of activity
  - time off school or work
- current medication:
  - regimen
  - compliance
  - technique
- measure:
  - height (children)
  - weight
  - PEFR (NB meters are now prescribable)
- reinforce advice re:
  - smoking (patients and parents)
  - exercise
  - weight
- reinforce education:
  - understanding of asthma
  - PEFR monitoring
  - effective inhaler technique
  - what to do in an acute attack
  - appropriate written back-up (eg Asthma Society leaflets and practice handouts)

Follow-up arranged

- Initial appointment:
  - review 1- or 2-weekly until controlled then 3-month review
  - annual review if in 'mild' group
  - 6-monthly review if in 'severe/moderate' group

PEFR Meters to be prescribed for all patients on inhaled steroids, and for other patients at doctors'/nurses' discretion.

After considerable background research, the protocol for the management of asthma was compiled very explicitly by the general practitioner according to age and severity of attacks; it is far too complex to include in detail here. To ensure effectiveness, audit was built into the protocol as a reassessment of the baseline audit after two years, with the possibility of a patient-satisfaction questionnaire.

The project was now complete, and the primary health care team members presented their work in the form of a proposal for discussion by partners and other members of the practice team at an educational breakfast meeting for eventual agreement to implement as practice policy. The four people who developed the protocol remain highly committed and actively involved in the care of asthma patients. They and other clinical personnel have further developed their specialized skills by attending courses for their continued education and to promote the level of expertise within the practice to provide a high quality service.

Almost two years on, in accordance with the protocol and in response to changes in health promotion funding, the practice manager is co-ordinating audit to complete the cycle. The audit will identify sources of information and people with the skills necessary to collect and analyse it to form the basis of discussion with the clinicians, who will review how well the practice adheres to the protocol and assess the need to improve the outcome of patient care in the light of the results. The same baseline data will be collected for direct comparison with the original figures.

[Extracts from the Asthma Protocol and Audit appear by kind permission of Dr P. E. Colyer of Claremont Surgery, Maidenhead.]

Asthma management is one aspect of preventive patient care; diabetes is the other chronic disease funded for primary care under Health Promotion Band 3. There is ample literature widely available to aid an approach to audit, and to help set realistic standards against which to measure quality of care. FHSAs specifically require data in support of applications for funding under Bands 1–3, but, though imposed externally and essential as a means to maximize income, practices will benefit from this opportunity to compare performance against their own objectives, and against standards attained both locally and nationally. A team approach to establishing protocols and audit is a learning experience in its own right, and a valuable educational tool in training.

9 Managing Money

Introduction: the practice manager as financial controller

ONE of the more important tasks of the practice manager is the control of the finances of the practice, ensuring that these are run in an efficient and systematic manner, maximizing the practice income, keeping a control on expenditure and hence increasing the profitability of the practice, not only for the benefit of the doctors but hopefully for the practice manager herself.

In these next sections we will look at several aspects of the manager's role as the financial controller of the practice. If one makes an analogy with the small limited trading company, the role is roughly equivalent to that of company secretary or finance director. It is one of huge responsibility; the modern medical practice may well have a turnover running into several hundred thousands of pounds. Practices with a turnover in excess of a million pounds are now becoming relatively common-place. This responsibility has increased following the introduction of fundholding to practices.

We do not consider here the personal aspects of general practice as they affect the doctors and partners themselves. Thus the subject of personal income tax, pensions and retirement, personal financing, etc. are not covered (and should be read in their proper context in the book *Making Sense of Practice Finance*, Second Edition by John Dean, published by Radcliffe Medical Press).

It is also essential that, having read this book and attended the courses, you keep your knowledge up to date.

Some of the manager's duties will concern employment; the hiring and firing of staff; payment of wages, etc. This will involve calculation of wages and salaries, a knowledge of PAYE and Class I National Insurance and this is described in that section.

One of the prime arts of management is the successful delegation of responsibility and the manager in general practice must be prepared to, where necessary, ensure that at least some part of her workload is delegated to more junior staff, whom it will be more cost effective to employ for that purpose.

Profitability and how to ensure it

General practice is a business, just as that of the dentist or the chemist or, outside the health care field, the normal conventional trader who buys goods and sells them for profit. They all have one thing in common: the profitable business will normally be the efficient one, and vice versa, although, of course, there is not necessarily a complete correlation between efficiency and the quality of patient care. In general medical practice this can be readily seen by those of us who have the opportunity to compare practices. It is by no means unusual to find two apparently identical practices, with similar numbers of patients and practising from very similar catchment areas, offering the same type of service and with similar numbers of partners, generating entirely different levels of income.

These discrepancies in income levels from general practice are both numerous and legendary. On the one hand, one may find a highly efficient dispensing practice, with numbers of outside appointments; probably some private patient work, with maximum staff levels, and the partners earning incomes in excess of £60 000 per annum. This will be a highly efficient business operation, with the partners all taking a share of responsibility for administration and the practice manager dealing with the day-to-day running of the practice, leaving the doctors largely to concentrate on their clinical duties to the ultimate benefit of patients.

At the other end of the scale, one comes across an apparently similar practice, with the partners having little interest in administration, probably operating on a shoestring with two or three part-time receptionists, little attention being made to maximize item-of-service claims and with a general air of decay and lack of attention. In this practice the partners may well earn no more than £20 000 – far less than even the intended average remuneration in general practice.

Although these are two extreme cases and are merely quoted to illustrate the point, they are by no means untypical of the situation in general practice today. It is often the quality of the practice manager who makes such a difference between two such examples.

If, then, it is accepted that efficiency equals profitability, how can you assure this efficiency and hence maximize the practice profits? For financial efficiency, a number of criteria are basic and necessary:

1 maximization of income from item-of-service fees;
2 achievement of targets;
3 an efficient system for the claiming of direct refunds
4 an adequate level of income from non-FHSA sources (*see* p. 162)
5 an economic cost structure, including up-to-date budgeting techniques (*see* 'Control of outgoings');
6 an effective bookkeeping system (*see* 'Basic bookkeeping');

7   a proper control of cash flow, including drawings systems (*see* 'Systems of drawings');
8   an interest and affinity with finance and administration by some or all of the partners.

These eight criteria will not automatically and of themselves create a highly profitable practice where none previously existed, but they will go a great deal of the way towards achieving it and give a foundation upon which to build.

Self-employment and the independent contractor status

The GP is a self-employed businessman, just as is his fellow professional, the solicitor or the architect, or the man running the high street shop. Unfortunately many doctors, starting their careers as they do as employees of a hospital authority, never see themselves as truly self-employed in every sense of the word, looking upon themselves as employees either of their practice or the health authority. This is far from being the case; the jealously-guarded status of the GP (and his colleague in the dental service) as independent contractors dates back to the formation of the NHS in 1948, when the status was negotiated on GPs' behalf and, apart from isolated occasions over the years when it has seriously been questioned, has stood the test of time.

This section has described what the term 'independent contractor' means. Why is it financially beneficial for the GPs? Let us have a look at this in some detail (*see* Box 9.1).

The advantages

A secured source of income

Unlike his colleagues in other professions, the NHS GP does not have to go out and look for clients (or, in his case, patients); they will come to him and he will normally have little difficulty, unless there is something radically wrong with his practice, in maintaining a standard list size. Indeed, in certain expanding areas, the list may increase at a fairly steady rate and the number of partners in the practice will normally be geared to such factors as the list size in order to ensure an adequate per capita level of income.

The receipt of a regular cheque at the end of each month and each quarter will help to ensure an even cash flow throughout the practice and the GP is saved the time and expense, which is common in other businesses, of having

---

Box 9.1:   The NHS GP as independent contractor

Advantages

Schedule D tax status
Occupational pension scheme
Freedom from fee collection
No top limit on earnings
Security of regular income

Obligations

Income enhancement by successful claims system
Necessity for running an efficient business
Desirability of efficient accounting records
Requirement to employ ancillary staff

---

to run complex credit control systems in order to ensure that bills are paid within a reasonable period.

Direct and indirect refunds of expenses

The manner in which refunds of expenditure are made, either by direct payment from the FHSA or by the system of indirect refund of expenses through the Review Body Award, is unique to general practice.

Pensions and superannuation

The NHS superannuation scheme, with proper advice, will give the GP an adequate income and lump sum on retirement. As a result of highly successful negotiations over the years, this has built-in factors such as dynamizing; index-linking; death in service benefits and other matters which are not normally found elsewhere.

Doctors (and their dentist colleagues) are the only people in the country who are both self-employed and members of an occupational pension scheme, in itself an advantage which can carry even further opportunities of enhancing their retirement income.

Taxation

GPs have the facility of being able to pay income tax under Schedule 'D', rather than by the Schedule 'E' status of an employee. The manner in which the respective tax schedules are administered ensures that the GP is considerably better off financially through paying tax as a self-employed professional.

This advantage will be moderated (but will by no means disappear) on the introduction of the current year basis of assessment from 1997/98.

The disadvantages

On the other hand, there are disadvantages as well. One rarely finds in this world that advantages of the nature outlined above are obtained without obligations in return and so it is with GPs.

Outside control of one's income

Just as the GP has a large element of security of his income, so he must accept the fact that, to a large degree, this is determined by an outside body, ie the Review Body. Again, this bears little comparison with his outside professional colleagues who are able to sell their own services at whatever fee they consider reasonable and economic, dependent only upon competition and market forces. The typical GP, excepting the relatively modest extra income he may obtain from non-NHS sources, is unable to do this and to a large degree is dependent on the annual remuneration award to determine the level of his income.

Control of staff

He will be responsible for the staffing of his surgery; hiring and firing of employees, calculation of salaries and all that this implies. Many GPs find themselves unable to deal adequately with staffing problems and this should ideally be delegated to the practice manager.

The responsibility of running a business

Most GPs experience continual difficulty, not only in running the business operation of their practice, but in the necessary contact they will have from time to time with other professions, such as accountants, lawyers, bank managers, etc. Without a proper business training they find themselves at a considerable disadvantage and in extreme cases it is not unknown for a young GP to seek to continue his career elsewhere, rather than subjecting himself to pressures of this nature.

In the properly organized general practice, an efficient and capable practice manager will take most, if not all, of these burdens from the shoulders of her doctors.

The Red Book and levels of fee income

The practice manager who wishes to take her duties seriously and to act in the best interest of her doctors, should familiarize herself as best she can with the Statement of Fees and Allowances (SFA) – known universally as 'The Red Book'. Supplied to all GPs in practice, the Red Book is the authoritative work on practice finance. Reference should be sought there for interpretation of any questions on practice finance.

The Red Book is a mine of information and a fully up-to-date amended copy should be available in every surgery. FHSAs issue amendments at fairly regular intervals throughout the year and care should be taken to see that the Red Book is always kept up-to-date for readily obtainable information. It has to be said, however, that it is not perhaps the most readable document. Fortunately, there are a supply of booklets which interpret the Red Book and again the conscientious practice manager should ensure that she keeps up-to-date with developments as they arise.

Making Sense of the Red Book, Second Edition, edited by John Chisholm and published by Radcliffe Medical Press, explains fees and allowances in a rather more readable form.

Fees and allowances payable to GPs are calculated each year and included in the annual Review Body Award.

What is far less often appreciated is the basis upon which intended remuneration levels are calculated. Each year the Review Body conducts a statistical sampling process, based upon practice accounts submitted to the Inland Revenue for income tax purposes. The accounts used in this review are restricted; at best they exclude any accounts not ending within the March quarter of each year; accounts prepared on a cash basis and those from practices in Northern Ireland are excluded also. This sampling process, not unlike a 'Gallup Poll' principle, extracts information from a variety of practices selected at random from these accounts available to the Inland Revenue. From this is prepared a calculation of expenses which in turn are converted to an average for a typical practice, and this then includes the element of indirect expenses refund included within GPs' remuneration.

It follows from this process that it is very much to the advantage of GPs as a whole that their accounts show the true level of their expenditure. In all too many cases, accounts are prepared and submitted which show expenditure 'netted-out' against the direct refunds received, so that either a nil or very small figure is included in those accounts. This is not acceptable; clear and precise instructions are included in the Red Book and the quotations of these are set out in the following paragraphs:

Drugs and appliances	para 44.12
Rent and rates:	para 51.36

Ancillary staff: para 52.21
Doctors in health care: para 53.4

The same principle also applies to presentation in accounts of the fundholding management allowance. Accountants preparing annual statements of account for GPs should understand and implement these requirements.

The generation of NHS income

As we have seen, ensuring the maximum level of profitability of the practice is one of the prime duties of a successful practice manager. She must be prepared, either herself or by suitable delegation, to ensure that:

1 the doctors are available to perform required levels of work for which the practice will receive payment;
2 a charge is made for such work, either NHS or private; and
3 payment is received for the work done within a reasonable period.

Let us now look at the main types of income which the practice can reasonably expect to receive from NHS sources and the means by which these are paid.

Practice allowances

The full Basic Practice Allowance (BPA) is dependent upon a number of factors applying:

1 that the GP is a principal in his practice;
2 that the practice has an average of at least 1200 patients on each partner's list, otherwise a reduced allowance will be paid, but not to partners with less than 400 patients unless in an 'inducement' area;
3 in a partnership, he receives not less than one-third of the remuneration of the highest paid partner (there are variations for part-time partners); and
4 the GP works at least 26 hours per week on surgeries, visits, etc.

Proportionately lower rates of BPA will be paid in respect of part-time GPs and job-sharers.

Postgraduate Education Allowance

GPs have to submit evidence to their FHSA or Health Board of having attended an average of five days a year over the past five years. This will be phased in over the first five years. Courses are approved by Regional Advisers and there must be at least two under each of the headings:

Health promotion
Disease management
Service management

The Department of Health has ruled that six hours will be equivalent to one day and there will be no half hours. There is now no claim for expenses as these are included in the allowance.

Seniority payments

These are paid in respect of years spent in practice:

First stage: registered 11 years: principal 7 years
Second stage: registered 18 years: principal 14 years
Third stage: registered 25 years: principal 21 years.

Capitation fees

This is a major proportion of total NHS income—some 63% on average. Higher fees are paid for the elderly. GPs are expected to offer patients over 75 at least one home visit annually and an assessment, for this enhanced capitation fee to be paid.

This forms an important part of income and it will be necessary to ensure that payment is received each quarter for patients who move into this age group.

Registration fees. A capitation fee is paid for all patients over five years newly registering with a practice upon which certain procedures are carried out. These have to be done within three months of the patient joining the practice and payment will be made at the end of each quarter. It is essential to have a system for ensuring an appointment for all new registrations as soon as possible and within the same quarter if possible.

Childhood surveillance fees. GPs who are suitably trained and who are on the Child Surveillance List maintained by the FHSA are paid a special capitation fee for each child registered. GPs on the list will be able to offer the service to patients registered with their partners as well. Payments are made quarterly.

Minor surgery

To claim a fee for this work, a GP must be included in the FHSA's Minor Surgery List. It is paid for minor surgery sessions provided for his or her own patients or those of partners or group members.

No more than three payments can be made to a GP in the same quarter, except that, if the GP is in a partnership or group practice, more payments may be claimed provided that the total number paid in any quarter does not exceed three times the number of partners or members of the group on the medical list on the first day of that quarter.

What is a session?

A session consists of five surgical procedures; they may be performed either in a single clinic or on separate occasions during the same quarter. Procedures will count towards a session if they meet the following criteria:

- they are included in this list:

Injections	intra articular
	peri articular
	varicose veins
	haemorrhoids
Aspirations	joints
	cysts
	bursae
	hydrocele
Incisions	abscesses
	cysts
	thrombosed piles
Excisions	sebaceous cysts
	lipomata
	skin lesions for histology
	intradermal naevi, papillomata, dermatofibromata and similar conditions
	warts
	removal of toe nails (partial and complete)
Curette cautery and cryocautery	warts and verrucae
	other skin lesions, eg molluscum contagiosum
Other	removal of foreign bodies
	nasal cautery

- they are performed by a doctor on the FHSA's Minor Surgery List
- any other person assisting in a procedure is suitably trained or experienced for the task.

Minor surgery list

A doctor who wants to perform minor surgery should apply to the FHSA for inclusion on the Minor Surgery List. The qualifying criteria are specified in the Regulations.

How to claim payment

Claims should be made on form FP/MS which records basic information about the patient's doctor, the doctor carrying out the procedure and the date and type of procedure. FHSAs check the validity of claims.

Item of service fees

There is no other single heading of income on which a GP's profitability level depends as much as on the efficient claiming of item of service fees. These are, in total, intended to account for 16% of a GP's income. The 1992–3 returned averages for England and Wales showed that the average fees per patient amounted to £4.48.

Many practices achieve higher rates, usually as a result of a busy location; for instance, one would expect practices in holiday resorts to have a much higher than average incidence of temporary resident fees, whereas those in rural backwaters are likely to have below average returns from maternity and family planning fees. Taken as a whole, the average is nevertheless a useful means of judging the financial efficiency of a practice and can act as a stimulus for generating higher levels of income than may previously have been possible.

- Item of service fees are paid for:
- night visits
- maternity medical services (MMS)
- emergency treatment and immediately necessary treatment
- contraceptive services
- temporary residents
- adult vaccinations and immunizations
- anaesthetization or arrest of dental haemorrhage.

Night visits

A GP is paid a fee for each visit requested and made between the hours of 10 pm and 8 am to a patient who is:

1 on his list of patients, *or*
2 a temporary resident, *or*

3   a woman for whom he has undertaken to provide MMS, provided the
    visit is related to these.

A fee is also paid if the GP provides treatment (eg minor surgery) in the surgery
in the patient's interests. If care is given in a treatment room of a GP hospital,
the fee is paid only if the GP is not on duty or on call for the hospital at the
time and the request for the treatment has not come from the hospital.
However, if the GP visits the patient in a hospital to provide MMS, a night
visit fee is paid if he holds an appointment at the hospital, but was not on
duty at the time, or if he does not hold such an appointment in respect of
MMS.
    A higher fee is payable if:

• the GP with whom the patient is registered makes the visit personally, *or*
• the visit is made by a partner or another GP from the group practice, *or*
• the visit is made by an assistant employed by a member of the partnership
  or group, *or*
• the visit is made by a regular locum or deputy employed by the partnership
  or group, provided the FHSA has been previously notified of the employment, *or*
• the visit is made by a trainee GP employed by the partnership or group,
  or
• the GP is single-handed or in a group practice or partnership, and is part
  of a local non-commercial rota which includes GPs outside the group or
  partnership who have agreed to provide out-of-hours cover for each other;
  they may also be single-handed or working in a group, but their number
  must not exceed 10. The FHSA needs to be informed of the details of these
  arrangements.

In all other cases, a lower fee is payable to the GP with whom the patient
requiring the visit is registered.

Maternity medical services (MMS)

A full MMS fee is paid to GPs who provide a comprehensive service during
the pregnancy of a patient, including the confinement and postnatal period.
In addition, a full postnatal examination at or about six weeks after confinement, and in any event no later than 12 weeks afterwards, must be carried
out. The full fee is payable provided that the GP accepts his patient's
application to receive these services, and that the application is accepted no
less than six weeks before the date of confinement.
    The higher rate MMS fee is paid only to GPs included on the Obstetric
List.
    The full criteria for payment under this scheme are set out in paragraph
31 of the SFA.

Emergency treatment

When a GP on the medical list of an FHSA is called upon, through accident or emergency, to treat a person neither on his own list nor on that of a partner, a fee should be paid for this emergency treatment. The detailed arrangements for payment of such fees are set out in paragraph 33 of the SFA.

Contraceptive services

An annual fee is payable under this heading if a GP accepts a patient, gives advice, and undertakes examinations and prescribes drugs or other aids as necessary. The fee is also payable if the GP takes steps to determine the patient's choice and accepts responsibility for any necessary after-care treatment. An intrauterine device fee is payable for services given in the 12 months commencing from the date of application to fit such a device.

Detailed conditions for payment of fees for contraceptive services are set out in paragraph 29 of the SFA.

Temporary residents

If a GP treats a patient resident in the area on a temporary basis, who is not on his own list, a fee will be paid: at a lower level if the patient expects to remain in the district for 15 days or less; or at a higher level if the patient expects to remain in the district for more than 15 days. In order to be considered as a temporary resident for this purpose, the patient must remain in the area for more than 24 hours. Separate regulations apply with regard to persons resident in holiday camps.

Detailed arrangements for payment of this fee are set out in paragraph 32 of the SFA.

Adult vaccinations and immunizations

Fees are payable for adult vaccinations or immunizations (or any ineligible for target payments) provided the patient is on the GP's own list or that of his partner, or is eligible for treatment as a temporary resident.

Target payments are made for childhood immunizations and pre-school boosters.

The regulations for payment of fees are complex as they are for treatment given to safeguard against certain conditions on an opportunistic basis. Full details are set out in paragraph 27 of the SFA.

Anaesthetization/dental haemorrhage arrest

In certain circumstances GPs may be called upon to act as anaesthetists or to arrest a dental haemorrhage. Whilst in many practices this will occur infrequently, GPs should be aware of the relevant fees. Detailed arrangements are set out in paragraph 34 and 35 of the SFA.

Claiming the correct fees and allowances

The NHS GPs' remuneration system is said to be the most complex in the world. It takes several hundred pages of the Regulations and the SFA to define with precision how a GP should be paid. Every practice should ensure that it is claiming the correct fees and allowances; otherwise it will lose out on its remuneration. On the other hand, no claim must be made, whether knowingly or unknowingly, for a fee or allowance to which a GP or practice is not eligible. A false or improper claim can lead to very serious consequences; FHSAs have not hesitated to instigate criminal prosecutions against GPs who have made such claims.

Target payments

Cervical cytology

GPs are no longer paid item of service fees for cervical cytology tests; instead payment is based on a system of target payments reflecting levels of uptake.

Eligibility

A GP will receive a target payment at the higher rate if, on the first day of each quarter, at least 80% of the eligible women on his or her list, aged between 25 and 64 (21 and 60 in Scotland), have had an adequate smear (taken by any source) during a period of 5.5 years preceding the claim. Women aged 25 to 64 are defined as those born between the second day of the same quarter 65 years earlier and the first day of the quarter 40 years later. For example, on 1 October 1993, the target population of women includes those born between 2 October 1928 and 1 October 1968.

A GP will be paid a target payment at the lower rate if at least 50% of the eligible women on the partnership list have had an adequate test.

When the scheme was initially proposed, target payments were to be calculated on an individual basis for each doctor, relating solely to the women registered on his or her list. However, the scheme was subsequently modified so that target payments were calculated on a partnership basis.

The actual payment depends on the number of eligible patients, compared with those on the list of the average GP, and the number of adequate smears taken as part of general medical services as opposed to those done in DHA or private clinics.

Who is excluded from the target calculation?

Women who have had hysterectomies involving the complete removal of the cervix are excluded from the total number of women on the list when calculating coverage. GPs should notify their FHSA of the number of women in the age group who have had hysterectomies, and the number of those women who have had an adequate smear in the preceding 5.5 years, and should inform it of any new cases. No other categories of women are excluded from the calculation.

Maximum sum payable

The maximum sum payable to a GP depends on the number of eligible women aged between 25 and 64 on the partnership list, compared with the average number of such women. The average number is calculated by multiplying 430 (the number of eligible women on the average GPs' list) by the number of partners. The maximum sum payable is therefore:

$$\frac{\text{number of eligible women on partnership list}}{430 \times \text{number of partners}} \times \frac{\text{maximum sum payable}}{\text{to the average GP}}$$

Calculating the payment

The GP is eligible for the whole of the relevant payment if at least 80%, or 50% for the lower target, of the eligible women have had adequate smear tests carried out by GPs as part of general medical services.

The smear test may have been undertaken by other doctors in the partnership or other GPs, for example if the woman was registered with another practice before joining the current GP's list. As long as the tests were adequate and carried out as part of general medical services, they are included. However, tests taken by a GP as part of work for which payment by a health authority or another source is received are excluded.

If any smears are repeated during the 5.5 year period, an adequate smear taken by a GP will take precedence over one taken by any other source for the purpose of calculating payments.

If the target is reached but the number of adequate smear tests carried out by GPs as part of general medical services is below the target number, the maximum payment is scaled down. The GP is paid that proportion of the maximum which the number of adequate tests hold to the target number.

Examples

The following two examples illustrate the target calculation and payment system.

Example 1: four-partner practice

Target calculation
Total number of eligible women aged 25–64
(hysterectomies excluded)   = 1440

Total number of women who have had an adequate smear
in the preceding 5.5 years   = 1200

$\dfrac{1200}{1440} \times 83.3\%$

Higher target payment is achieved. The number of smears required to reach the higher target (the target number) is 1152 (80% of 1440).

Calculation of maximum sum payable

$$\text{Maximum sum payable} = \frac{1440 \text{ (number of eligible women on partnership list)}}{430 \text{ (number of eligible women on average list)} \times 4 \text{ (number of partners)}} \times \text{Maximum sum payable for the average practitoner (80\% level)}$$

Calculation of payment
Total number of adequate smears = 1200
of which 800 done by GP or partner
      160 done by another GP
      200 done by DHA
       40 done privately.

Therefore 960 were undertaken under general medical services.

$\text{Maximum sum payable} \times \dfrac{960}{1152} = \text{actual payment to each partner}$

Example 2: three-partner practice

Target calculation
Total number of eligible women aged 25–64
(hysterectomies excluded)   = 600

Total number of women who have had an adequate smear
in the preceding 5.5 years   = 330

$$\frac{330}{600} = 55\%$$

Lower target payment is achieved. The number of smears required to reach the lower target (the target number) is 300 (50% of 600).

Calculation of maximum sum payable

$$\text{Maximum sum payable} = \frac{600}{430 \times 3} \times \begin{array}{c} \text{maximum sum payable for} \\ \text{the average practitioner} \\ \text{(50\% level)} \end{array}$$

Calculation of payment
Total number of adequate smears = 330
of which 240 done by GP or partner
        45 done by another GP
        30 done by DHA
        15 done privately.

Therefore 285 were undertaken under general medical services.

$$\text{Maximum sum payable} \times \frac{285}{300} = \text{actual payment to each partner}$$

By April 1994 all FHSAs should have sufficient data on their computer systems to calculate entitlement to payments. Meanwhile, FHSAs may apportion tests of unclear origin in proportion to the known proportion of tests carried out by a GP for women on his or her list. For example, if the source of 12 tests is unclear and a GP has been responsible for taking the tests of 150 women on his or her eligible list of 192, then $\frac{150}{180} \times 12$, ie 10, of the unclear source tests will be allowed for payment.

An FHSA will also accept until 1994 information based on a GP's own records; GPs should use form FP/TCC to claim if the evidence from practice records indicates that a target has been reached. The validity of the claim may be checked by the FHSA.

Immunization for children aged two and under

A target payment system has replaced the previous individual payments for each immunization provided to children under the age of two.

Eligibility

A GP is eligible for a higher rate target payment if, on the first day of a quarter, the number of courses completed in each of the following groups of immunizations amounts on average to 90% of the number needed to achieve full immunization of all children aged two on his or her list. For the purpose of calculation, children aged two are defined as those born between the second day of the same quarter three years earlier and the first day of the corresponding quarter one year later, inclusive. For example, on 1 October 1993, the target population of children includes those born between 2 October 1990 and 1 October 1991.

Group one		Group two	Group three	
Diptheria		Pertussis 3 doses	Measles	1 dose
Tetanus	3 doses		OR	
Poliomyelitis			Measles	
			Mumps	3 doses
			Rubella	

A GP will be eligible for a lower rate target payment if the average of courses completed amounts to 70% of the number needed for full immunization.

When the scheme was first proposed, payment was to be based on an individual GP's list; the scheme was subsequently modified so that target payments were calculated on a partnership basis.

Maximum sum payable

The maximum sum payable depends on the number of children aged two on the partnership list, compared with the average number.

The average number is calculated by multiplying 22 (the number of children aged two on the average GP's list) by the number of partners. The maximum sum payable is therefore:

$$\frac{\text{number of children aged two on partnership list}}{22 \times \text{number of partners}} \times \begin{array}{c}\text{maximum sum}\\ \text{payable to}\\ \text{average GP}\end{array}$$

Calculating the payment

The proportion of the payment due to the GP depends on the number of courses of immunization completed by doctors as part of general medical services as opposed to those completed elsewhere, for example at health authority clinics.

A course completed by other GPs (inside or outside the partnership) as part of general medical services will count towards the payment of the doctor making the claim. This means that, if a child who has had all the completing doses moves and registers with another practice, the new practice can count that child towards its target payment even though it provided none of the immunizations.

A course will be considered as being completed by a GP as part of general medical services if he or she gives the final immunization needed to complete cover for the diseases in that group. Thus in group one the completing immunization will be the third poliomyelitis, if the child has also had three doses of diptheria and tetanus vaccine.

Method of calculation

The first step is to decide how many completing immunizations are needed to reach a target. Twenty children have 60 immunization groups; so 42 completing immunizations would be required to reach the 70% target, and 54 for the 90% target. If the calculation results in a fraction, the target will be rounded to the nearest integer (0.5 being rounded down).

Secondly, it is necessary to decide whether a target has been reached by adding the numbers of completing immunizations carried out in each of the three groups. Thus, completing immunizations in excess of the target number in one group can top up the number in another group.

Thirdly, if a target has been achieved, it is necessary to calculate the maximum sum payable, comparing the actual number of eligible children with the average number.

Fourthly, it is necessary to count the number of completing immunizations carried out by GPs as part of general medical services for the three immunization groups, so that the appropriate proportion of the maximum sum payable can be calculated. Only one completing immunization per child can be counted for each group. Where the number of completing immunizations in each group done by GPs as part of general medical services is greater than the number of children needed to reach the target level, the latter figure is counted. For example, if a partnership has 40 children aged two on its list, 32 have completed their immunizations in each of the three groups, and all the completing doses were given by GPs, then the 70% target has been reached. As the 70% target number is 28 children who have had completing immunizations, only 28 count towards the work done by GPs in each group.

Therefore, the number of completing immunizations done by GPs is regarded as 28 + 28 + 28 = 84 (= 100% of the number needed to reach the 70% target).

Finally, the actual amount payable is then calculated by multiplying the maximum sum payable by the number of completing immunizations done as part of general medical services for the three groups added together, counted in the manner described in the previous paragraph, and dividing by the number necessary to achieve the appropriate percentage cover. As there are three groups, the number necessary to achieve the target is the appropriate percentage of three times the number of children concerned.

If a GP works for another body such as a health authority, any immunization carried out as part of this other contract will not count towards payment. Work done by employed or attached staff at the direction of a GP as part of general medical services is, however, counted for payment.

How to claim

Claims should be made on form PT/TC1 no later than four months after the date to which the claim relates. GPs should report details of all immunizations to the appropriate health authorities and also inform the FHSA of any health authority appointments they hold which involve immunization work.

Example: six-partner practice

On the first day of the quarter a partnership of 6 doctors has 120 children aged two on its list. All 120 have had complete courses of immunizations against diptheria, tetanus and poliomyelitis. Sixty of the completing immunizations were given by the GP's own practice, 30 by another GP practice and 30 by a DHA clinic.

Ninety of the children have had complete courses of immunization against pertussis. Of these 48 were given by the GP's own practice, none by another GP practice and 42 by a DHA clinic.

Seventy-two of the children have been immunized against measles, mumps and rubella. Of these courses, 30 were given by the GP's own practice, 12 by another GP practice and 30 by a DHA clinic.

Step one: How many completing immunizations are needed to reach a target?
One-hundred-and-twenty children have a maximum of 360 completing immunizations.
The 70% target requires 252 completing immunizations.
The 90% target requires 324 completing immunizations.

Step two: Has a target been reached?

Group 1 (DT and P)	120
Group 2 (Pertussis)	90
Group 3 (MMR)	72
Total	282

The 70% target has been reached.

Step three: What is the maximun sum payable?

$$\frac{120}{22 \times 6} \times \begin{array}{c} \text{maximum sum payable to} \\ \text{GP with an average list} \end{array} = \text{maximum sum payable}$$

Step four: What proportion of the work needed to reach the target was done by GPs as part of general medical services?

Group 1	GP's own practice	60
	Another GP	30
	Total	90

but since 70% = 84 immunizations, this is treated as 84

Group 2	GP's own practice	48
	Another GP	0
	Total	48

Group 3	GP's own practice	30
	Another GP	12
	Total	42

Group 1	84
Group 2	48
Group 3	42
Total of completing doses regarded as carried out by GPs	174

Step five: How much is the payment?

Number of completing immunizations regarded as given by GPs = 174

Number of completing immunizations needed to reach 70% = 252

Payment per partner $= \dfrac{174}{252} \times$ maximun sum payable for 70% target

Pre-school boosters for children aged five and under

Just as target payments are available for immunization of children aged two and under, they are also paid for pre-school boosters for children aged five and under.

Eligibility

A GP is eligible for a target payment at the higher rate if, on the first day of each quarter, 90% of the children on the partnership list who are aged five have had reinforcing doses of diptheria, tetanus and polio immunizations. Children aged five are defined as those born between the second day of the same quarter six years earlier and the first day of the quarter a year later. For example, on 1 October 1993, the target population of children includes those born between 2 October 1987 and 1 October 1988.

If 70% of the children under five have reinforcing doses then a target payment at the lower rate will be made. The payment to be made will depend on the number of eligible patients, compared with the average number, and on the number of boosters given by GPs as opposed to those given by others. A child will only be considered as fully immunized if he or she has received booster doses of all three vaccines. One or two vaccines will not count.

Maximum sum payable

The number of children aged five on the partnership list compared to an average list will determine the maximum sum payable. The average number is calculated by multiplying 22 (the number of children aged five on the average GP's list) by the number of partners. The maximum sum payable is therefore:

$$\frac{\text{number of children aged five on the partnership list}}{22 \times \text{number of partners}} \times \begin{array}{c} \text{maximum sum payable} \\ \text{to average GP} \end{array}$$

Calculating the payment

The amount payable depends on the level of cover achieved and the number of complete booster doses of immunizations given by GPs as part of general medical services. Those provided by other sources, for example health authority clinics, do not count. Boosters given by other GPs under general medical services – for example if a child is given the necessary boosters by a GP in one practice and then moves to another part of the country and registers with a new doctor – will be counted in the target calculation of the claiming

GP. The child will be counted towards the new GP's target levels and not those of the doctor who gave the boosters.

The first step in working out the payment to be made is to decide whether 90% or 70% of the total number of children have received booster doses for all three vaccines. In calculating the 90% or 70% target number, fractions will be rounded to the nearest integer (0.5 being rounded down). If a child does not have all three boosters at the same time, no account will be taken of them until all three boosters have been given. The booster will count as having been given by whoever gave the third booster dose.

Secondly, if a target is reached, the number of booster doses given as part of general medical services is counted so that the appropriate proportion of the maximum sum payable can be calculated.

Thirdly, the actual amount is calculated by multiplying the maximum sum payable by the number of booster doses given under general medical services, and dividing by the number of boosters necessary to achieve the appropriate percentage cover.

Work does not count as having been performed by a GP as part of general medical services if he or she immunizes children under a paid contract outside the GMS system. Work done by employed staff or attached staff under the direction of a GP as part of general medical services will, however, be counted.

How to claim

Claims should be made to the FHSA on form FP/TPB no later than four months after the date on which eligibility is assessed.

GPs are responsible for reporting all immunizations to the appropriate health authority as soon as they are given. This allows health authorities to provide GPs with information to help them in claiming payments.

GPs are also responsible for reporting to the FHSA any appointment that they hold with a health authority which includes providing pre-school boosters.

Health promotion payments

For many years, GPs have been involved in opportunistic health promotion, planned call and recall of patients for preventive care and the planned management of patients with chronic diseases. Until 1990, this work was undertaken as part of general medical services, without any specific payment or any additional funding; the profession was rewarded within average net remuneration.

However, the GP contract introduced on 1 April 1990 made health promotion a specific obligation under GPs' terms of service. GPs were obliged to give 'advice, where appropriate, to a patient in connection with the patient's general health, and in particular about the significance of diet, exercise, the use of tobacco, the consumption of alcohol and the misuse of drugs or solvents', as well as to offer 'consultations and, where appropriate, physical examinations for the purpose of . . . reducing the risk of disease or injury'.

In addition, GPs were able to claim fees for health promotion clinics. Well-person clinics, anti-smoking clinics, clinics for alcohol control, dietary advice, exercise counselling, stress management, heart disease prevention, and the care of patients with diabetes or asthma generally qualified for payment, and other clinics could also be submitted for approval by FHSAs. So long as the purpose of and arrangements for clinics were approved by the FHSA, there was no limit on the number of clinics for which GPs could claim.

A rapid growth in expenditure on clinics resulted: in 1990–1, £50 million was paid to GPs in Great Britain by way of health promotion clinic fees, in the second year of the scheme £73 million was paid out, and in the third year £80 million was claimed. Although collectively GPs were doing more and more work for the same total pool of money, individual GPs sought to maximize their own income by undertaking increasing numbers of clinics, and the level of activity only stopped climbing with the imposition of a moratorium on 1 July 1992. If a moratorium had not been imposed, there was every reason to suppose that the amount GPs were earning from health promotion clinics would have gone on increasing, with the result that GPs would have been paid less and less for the rest of their work. Indeed, the growth in health promotion clinics was a major factor in the destabilization of the GP remuneration system which occurred after the introduction of the 1990 contract.

This clinic activity was very unevenly distributed among practices, with no activity being recorded in many and substantial amounts in others. The distribution could not easily be explained by the needs of patients, and the problem was undoubtedly compounded by the application of differing approval criteria by different FHSAs and Health Boards. The profession collectively said that it felt cheapened and demoralized by, and cynical about, the operation of the clinic system, coupled with GP's obligation under the Regulations introduced in 1990 to offer a consultation to patients between the ages of 16 and 75 years who had not been seen in general practice within the preceding three years. There was thus considerable pressure for change in the contractual arrangements governing health promotion, and protracted negotiations were undertaken in order to achieve a new system, and to supersede the requirement for GPs to invite non-attenders for three-yearly checks.

The intention was to fashion a system with greater accountability, greater equitability and greater scientific validity, as well as greater professional freedom, recognizing in particular the value of opportunistic intervention. Both Government and profession wanted to see resources targeted on proven activities which would be of greatest benefit to patients. The negotiations took place within the framework set up by the White Paper *The Health of the Nation*, published in July 1992, and the equivalent Scottish and Welsh strategic guidance, and it was decided to focus health promotion activity on the prevention of coronary heart disease and stroke.

It was also seen that health promotion activities had to be appropriate to local needs and circumstances, and to reflect dialogue between FHSAs, LMCs and GPs. FHSAs and DHAs would need to make information available to practices on other relevant local health promotion activities, so that unnecessary duplication could be avoided.

The payment arrangements would need to encourage the wider availability to patients of consistent health promotion programmes, to produce a more equitable distribution of income to GPs, and to deliver a more predictable year-on-year allocation of resources to health promotion activities. It was therefore decided during the negotiating process that health promotion and chronic disease management should be paid for from a pool within a pool: within the total amount of money available for GPs' remuneration, a fixed sum should be set aside for these activities. The size of that pool was to be similar to the amount spent on clinics during the third year of their operation. Such an approach had the virtues of stopping further devaluation of the amount GPs were paid for the rest of their work (including the treatment of sick patients), of circumscribing the level of total health promotion activity, and of making it easier to resist the inclusion of additional activities in the work of GPs without the provision of new money to pay for them. Additionally, the risk of overpayments being made to the profession – which would then need to be clawed back under the Review Body's balancing arrangements – would be controlled by a system of annual bidding and fee adjustment.

Transitional arrangements and priorities reflecting local circumstances

Despite the concentration of the care programme on coronary heart disease, stroke, asthma and diabetes, and despite the intention to ensure that health promotion is appropriately and adequately resourced, the new scheme is also intended to allow the addressing of other locally agreed priorities, flowing either from central strategic intentions or from the identification of particular local needs. Many practices had already been undertaking worthwhile activity outside the scope of the core programme, and further developments should be encouraged when circumstances and resources permit.

In the first nine months of the new scheme's operation, from 1 July 1993 to 31 March 1994, transitional payments will be available to those practices offering a band three health promotion programme, which were earning more money under the previous health promotion clinic arrangements than they can now earn from band three activities and asthma and diabetes care programmes, so long as they are carrying out an approved transitional programme.

In the second year of the scheme, from 1 April 1994 to 31 March 1995, it is intended that money will be redeployed from the transitional fund, to fund new activity within the care programmes and to resource new and existing activity within locally agreed priorities, and by the third year of the scheme, the entire transitional fund will have been redeployed in that way.

Meanwhile, in the second year of the scheme, transitional payments will continue to be paid to practices which had been receiving them from the start of the new system, but at approximately half the rate paid in the first nine months.

Organization of programmes

Practices will have to apply for approval of their programmes on an annual basis, by 31 January each year, on form FP/HPP/1, and to report progress in their annual reports by 30 June. They also have to include mid-year summaries of their progress to date on form FP/HPP/2, with their applications for reapproval.

It is open to single-handed doctors and two doctor practices to collaborate with others to organize and offer a joint programme if they wish.

The information in the Red Book about health promotion and chronic disease management has been supplemented by extensive guidance for regional authorities, FHSAs, LMCs and practices, sent out by the Department of Health on 12 January 1993 (FHSL(93)3). The guidance emphasizes that the information required by FHSAs in order to determine whether the

---

Box 9.2: Consultation with the LMC

- Development of health promotion programmes in relation to *Health of the Nation* and strategic policy documents.
- Local factors relevant to programmes.
- Selection of priority groups.
- Level of coverage.
- Shared care arrangements for chronic disease management.
- Approach to borderline or unusual cases.

programme meets the Red Book criteria should not be excessive or repetitive. Many practices will have referred in their applications to protocols or guidelines already approved under the old clinic arrangements, or to readily available national clinical guidance.

FHSAs are required to consult LMCs on the way in which the guidance from the Department of Health is followed through locally. Such consultation is required on issues arising from *The Health of the Nation* and regional, DHA and FHSA strategies for meeting Health of the Nation targets which should be taken into account in developing health promotion programmes; on local factors relevant to the development of health promotion programmes, including the selection of priority groups; on the level of coverage to be expected, and whether variations from national guidance are justified by local circumstances; and on the shared care arrangements for chronic disease management. FHSAs may also consult LMCs on the approach to be adopted in relation to borderline or unusual cases (*see* Box 9.2).

The Department of Health is taking an active role centrally and through the regions, in order to promote the fair and consistent application of the new arrangements throughout the country, and is encouraging dialogue at regional level between NHS management and the profession about the framework, its implementation and any inconsistencies in interpretation.

Annual reports and information requirements

The move from health promotion clinics to health promotion programmes is founded on a more population-based approach to preventive care. Some basic information on the practice population is needed to underpin these programmes, and is to be summarized in annual reports. Many practices already hold such information, but for some it will be a new task; practices without computers face a particular challenge.

The contents of annual reports have therefore been rationalized; some previous requirements have been pruned, including information about premises, staffing and referrals, so as to eliminate duplication of data available elsewhere. The aim is to concentrate on information needed to support the new programmes, building on basic information supplied by all GPs on the health of their practice population.

Additional information will be expected from GPs offering health promotion or chronic disease management programmes, including a commentary indicating whether progress on coverage levels has been as expected, whether changes in the programme have been or will be required, what audit has been carried out, and whether joint working with other individuals or agencies has occurred.

The degree of detail in which practices compile information will be influenced by whether or not they are computerized, their computer's reporting capacity, and their own needs and interests. Rates of progress towards comprehensive information gathering will vary, and in the first year of the scheme it is acceptable for practices starting from a low base to demonstrate good progress, if they cannot meet the information requirements in full.

The detailed information requirements are defined in the Red Book, while the Departmental guidance suggests methods of presenting the data. In summary, information will be collected on a head count basis – the numbers of patients given advice, offered interventions etc – rather than an activity basis – the number of clinic sessions – and will be broken down by age and sex.

Other NHS income

In many practices, income is derived from NHS sources outside the main fees and allowances paid by the FHSA. Some of this additional income is likely to take the form of salaries and remuneration from local hospitals or other NHS institutions. In a partnership care must be taken to ensure that these are properly treated and that the allocation of such income between the partners is in accordance both with their wishes and with the provisions of the partnership deed.

One major problem which derives from this source of income is the deductions which may well be taken before the net fees are received. These deductions are likely to take the form of superannuation, income tax and probably national insurance. The practice accountant should be consulted as to exactly how these are to be charged both to the partners in whose name the positions are held, and through the partnership accounts so as to ensure fairness and equity between the partners. These problems do not arise in the case of sole practitioners, the income being wholly that of the GP concerned.

Non-NHS income

GPs are not restricted to earning their income from NHS sources and frequently they will go outside the NHS to earn a proportion of their income. In some cases this can be a relatively high proportion, particularly in 'police' practices and those living in an area which naturally attracts a high incidence of private patients.

In some practices a high source of earnings can result from retainers and annual fees paid by nursing homes, schools and commercial organizations for one or some of the partners acting as medical officer. It is wise to negotiate a realistic fee for this before the work is taken on and to have a suitable contract drawn up.

The typical practice, however, will receive a fairly steady source of income from insurance examinations and reports; cremation and sundry certificate fees. It will be seen in the section on petty cash exactly how this money is to be dealt with but care must be taken to see that it is properly recorded in the books of the practice, both to ensure again that each partner receives his proper share of the income but also so that it does not give rise to an enquiry into fees not returned for tax purposes.

The allocation of this income in medical partnerships can frequently be a problem. It is invariably advisable to have a rule that all income from medical sources, of whatever type, is to be aggregated with the partnership income and divided between the partners in agreed ratios. It is a ready-made source of friction between partners where some doctors retain part of their earnings, with their partners frequently feeling aggrieved at this not being included in the partnership pool of income.

Dispensing practices

In some cases practices will have the right to dispense drugs to patients on their lists. This is normally restricted to patients who live more than a mile from a chemist's shop. Those doctors who are able to do dispensing work of this nature have a steady source of additional income, the dispensing fees being paid out in accordance with scales in force from time to time. A practice of this nature will probably employ a qualified dispenser who can deal with the detailed work on the dispensing of drugs. They will make returns to the FHSA from time to time; the prescriptions will be priced and a refund will ultimately be made to the partnership for the cost of those drugs, plus the dispensing fee.

It is common for such refunds to be made two or even three months in arrears. However, in order to obtain maximum discount, it is probably necessary to pay the wholesale chemist at least monthly, so that the practice will need to have a fair measure of working capital in order to finance the stock of drugs which must be held at any given time. A great deal of the profitability from such practices derives from the generous discounts which are regularly made available to dispensing GPs.

Direct refunds

The practice will receive refunds in respect of rent (if it is a rented surgery), rates of various descriptions, ancillary staff and staff national insurance contributions. These recovery rates may be affected by cash limiting procedures imposed by the FHSA.

Where refunds of rates are claimed, care must again be taken to ensure that all refunds of such items as sewerage and water rates, drainage rates in certain areas and the like are also claimed. In some cases it will be possible to claim a refund of local authority refuse collection charges as well for the disposal of 'sharps'. In some urban areas, it may be possible to claim a refund of car parking contract charges paid to local authorities. Some practices lose thousands of pounds a year by not submitting these claims in a regular and efficient manner.

In addition to this and to the refunds of drugs described above, training practices must claim a refund of their trainee's salaries. Although not strictly speaking a refund, if doctors are away for reasons of sickness or on maternity leave, an allowance might be claimed in certain circumstances, which is intended to cover the cost of employing a locum.

Most FHSAs allocate non-fundholding practices an indicative staff salary budget to cover 70% of gross staff salaries plus 100% of the Employers NI contribution. There is a general shift towards a capitation based formula for funding, to be introduced over the next few years. This will rationalize the cash limited funding between all types of practices, whether fundholding or non-fundholding and include factors such as ethnicity, branch surgeries and areas of deprivation. It encourages practice managers to look carefully at their staffing structure and review each vacancy before recruiting automatically to replace like with like.

Leave advances

A great help to the cash flow of both the practice and the individual doctors is the claiming of the leave advance. This is 20% of the Basic Practice Allowance and should be claimed by submission of Form FP75 to the FHSA by 15 April each year.

Internal control questionnaire for medical practices

1 General accounting organization
(a) Are the accounting records maintained up-to-date and balanced monthly?
(b) Do the partners appear to take a direct and active interest in the financial affairs of the practice?
(c) Are there any systems of periodic financial reports or budgetary control?
(d) Are the personal funds and financial transactions of the partners completely segregated from the partnership?

2 Receipts
(a) Is the mail opened by the partners?
(b) Are sundry cash receipts separately recorded?
(c) Is money received banked intact?

3 Payments
(a) Are all payments made by cheque?
(b) Can cheques be signed only by the partners?
(c) Are cheques signed only when complete (i.e. not blank)?
(d) Is supporting documentation approved and cancelled by the partners when payment is made?
(e) Is supporting documentation properly filed, consecutively numbered and cross-referenced to the cash book?
(f) Are spoiled cheques retained?
(g) Are payments not made by cheque (e.g. standing orders) authorized only by the partners?
(h) Do the partners review the bank reconciliations?
(i) Is petty cash maintained on an imprest system?

4 Fees and debtors (for private patients)
(a) Are fee notes pre-numbered and all accounted for?
(b) Is a list of unpaid fees regularly reviewed by the partners?
(c) Are reminders sent to patients in respect of overdue fees?

5 Drawings
(a) Are partners' drawings paid regularly (e.g. monthly)?
(b) Do the calculations for regular drawings take account of tax reserves, disparities in allowances, etc.?
(c) Are the amounts of regular drawings periodically reviewed during the year in the light of practice income and any changes in profit sharing ratios?
(d) Are Class 2 National Insurance Contributions paid regularly by the partnership and debited to the partners' current accounts?

6 Wages and salaries
(a) Are employees taken on or dismissed only by the partners (or, where delegated, the practice manager)?
(b) Are references obtained in respect of new employees?
(c) Are PAYE and National Insurance deductions paid over monthly to the Collector of Taxes?

7 Fixed assets
(a) Are detailed records maintained of the assets owned by the practice?
(b) Are the partners aware of which assets are owned by the practice and which are owned by the individual partners?
(c) Are disposals and scrapping of assets authorized only by the partners?

8   Stock (for dispensing practices)
(a)   Are continuous stock records maintained?
(b)   Is stock physically counted periodically and reconciled to the stock
      records and dangerous drugs book?

Control of outgoings

We have had a look at means by which income can be maximized. However,
this is by no means the full story. In order to achieve maximum profitability,
some control must also be kept on outgoings and it is only by some sound
method of budgeting and constant cost control that the practice is run in as
economic a manner as possible.

One essential feature of the control of costs is the drawing up of a proper
expenditure budget, it is suggested by the practice manager and agreed by the
partners before the commencement of each financial year. For this it is
necessary to know the date to which the partnership's annual accounts are
prepared. This will normally be one of the conventional quarter days, i.e. 31
March, 30 June, 30 September or 31 December. Whichever date is used, the
budget should be formulated and agreed as soon as possible beforehand. It
may be that, following the completion of the practice accounts by the
accountant, which at its earliest cannot for practical reasons take place at less
than a few months after the end of each financial year, the budget will need
to be revised, but a close monthly check should be kept on expenditure and
if necessary checks and economies instituted.

It may be that there are exceptional items which cannot be controlled; for
instance, a partner may be required to take sickness or maternity leave which
involves the partnership in additional locum expenses. There may be unfor-
seen repairs required to the building or an exceptional increase in telephone
or heating charges, but it is normally possible to build in some leeway in the
budget to cater for these.

Table 9.1 illustrates a typical but simplified expenditure budget for a
training practice of five partners. This shows the annual budgeted cost; the
monthly actual and cumulative costs for the first two months of the year,
October and November 1994 and how it is possible to make a running check
of expenses by this means.

Before doing this it is important to specify which items of expenditure are
to be paid out of the partnership account and which are to be borne by the
individual partners personally. A number of items of expenditure may well
be paid by either of these means, depending on partnership policy. This
should be clearly specified beforehand and set out in precise terms in the
partnership deed so as to leave no room for misinterpretation. Such items
could well be:

Table 9.1   Expenditure budget.

Control Sheet: Year to 30 September 1994

	Annual budget cost (£)	October 1994		November 1994	
		Actual (£)	To date (£)	Actual (£)	To date (cumulative) (£)
Drugs and appliances	2000	—	—	100	100
Locum fees	3000	—	—	—	—
Deputizing	1000	50	50	50	100
Equipment hire	1500	200	200	150	350
NHS levies	500	—	—	—	—
Training costs	600	50	50	30	80
Books and Journals	100	—	—	20	20
Staff salaries (inc. NIC)	30 000	2500	2500	2350	4850
Trainees' salaries	15 000	1250	1250	1250	2500
Staff welfare	1000	100	100	50	150
Recruitment costs	500	—	—	80	80
Rates and water	5300	400	400	400	800
Light and heat	1500	—	—	150	150
Repairs and renewals	2000	500	500	100	600
Insurance premiums	800	—	—	200	200
Cleaning and laundry	2000	200	200	200	400
Garden expenses	500	50	50	20	70
Printing, stationery and postage	1800	500	500	200	700
Telephone	4800	500	500	200	700
Accountancy	4200	—	—	—	—
Bank charges	200	—	—	100	100
Legal charges	200	—	—	100	100
Sundry expenses	1500	200	200	100	100
TOTAL BUDGETED COSTS	80 000	6500	6500	5850	12 350

Partners' car expenses
Private telephone charges
Spouses' salaries, pensions, etc.
Medical subscriptions
Private accountancy fees

If these are to be borne individually by the partners they should not be included as items of expenditure in any practice budget.

If this applies, such items should ideally not be paid out of partnership funds. Although honour can be satisfied by charging these to the partners' current accounts, as merely an extra item of drawing, nevertheless this is likely to give rise to big inequalities between the partners at the end of each year, which must be balanced annually. It is therefore advised that such personal items of expenditure be paid by the partners out of their own bank accounts and not out of partnership funds.

Basic bookkeeping and accounts

General practice, is a business; probably a very big business. Even a small practice is likely to have a turnover running into six figures.

Were this a conventional business enterprise, it would likely as not employ skilled accounting staff to deal with its affairs and the problem of inadequate records would not apply. Doctors, however, are notoriously bad both at keeping their own personal records and those of their practices or partnerships.

Most doctors have had no financial training whatever. Yet on entering general practice they might well find themselves, within a relatively short period, equity partners in a medium-sized business enterprise, having to participate in any number of far-reaching decisions affecting the finances of themselves, their partners and their staff; employment and staffing; budgeting and controls; taxation, insurance, banking and investment.

It need hardly be said that such decisions as have to be taken regularly in all medical practices are virtually impossible without access to proper, well-maintained and comprehensive accounting records. Hopefully those records will be kept, or at the very least supervised, by a competent practice manager and they will form the basis of the practice's financial reporting facility. No true business decisions can be made without them.

One is frequently asked why records of this nature should be kept; why it could not all be kept by an accountant. The prime reasons for keeping such bookkeeping records are:

1   to identify items of income and to highlight means by which this can be maximized;
2   conversely, to keep a close watch on expenditure and through successful budgeting control costs economize;
3   by means of the above, to maximise profits and hence the income of the partners;
4   the partnership deed may well include a clause to the effect that 'proper bookkeeping records shall be kept';
5   records will be available in the event of enquiry by the Inland Revenue into the practice's affairs; and
6   a possible saving in accounting fees.

It is sometimes found that outside accountants keep the books of the practice but this will almost certainly cost the partners a great deal of unnecessary expense. Accountants' time is expensive and it is wholly uneconomic to have a professional person dealing with routine bookkeeping records of this nature.

One advantage not possessed by any other business, as we have seen, is the facility to recover some or all of the costs of employing ancillary staff and their national insurance contributions. This can be extended to include clerical staff such as bookkeepers and it obviously makes financial sense to employ one's own staff for this purpose rather than to use an accountant, whose fees will not only be expensive but will certainly not be recoverable, either wholly or partly from the FHSA, as well as including a 17.5% VAT charge.

Firstly let us look briefly at the type of bookkeeping records which should be kept.

Petty cash

The basic record for all cash transactions is the petty cash book, probably with the actual cash on hand on any given date being maintained in one or two petty cash boxes specifically used for that purpose. The maintenance of an efficient and well-regulated system of petty cash control and recording is an integral part of the practice's bookkeeping arrangements.

What exactly is meant by petty cash? It does of course mean coin of the realm and bank notes, either received by the practice from patients as fee income or available in the form of a float, from which sundry cash disbursements can be made. These two aspects of petty cash in the average general practice should be kept entirely distinct.

It cannot be too strongly emphasized that any fees received in cash, of whatever nature, for certificates, sundry other fees, and especially cremation fees should be properly accounted for and paid into the practice bank account without deduction.

The notion is incorrect (but nevertheless it persists) that these fees are in some way 'perks' which need not be accounted for and which the doctor is entitled to put into his pocket without paying tax on. Nothing could be further from the truth; these are the income from his profession and it is essential that they are fully accounted for, both for accountancy and taxation purposes.

There are some doctors who have had a rude shock recently by finding that, for instance, cremation fees have been traced by the Inspector of Taxes and that they are asked to pay tax upon them, for several years in arrears.

Cash receipts of this nature should always be collected together separately and paid to the practice bank periodically. Many practices retain such cash on hand in a separate tin for a period of, say, a week or a fortnight, or perhaps upon reaching a previously agreed sum.

A great deal will depend on the circumstances of the practice and the volume of fees received, but a policy once established should be strictly adhered to.

It is also recommended that a separate book be kept to record these sundry fees received, not only as a routine record but to enable the practice manager to check whether any given fee has been received. This could have a separate column for recording receipts of a non-fee nature and it is also suggested that a separate column be maintained for recording cremation fees. The actual cash should be collected in a separate cash tin retained for this purpose only, which is cleared fully when the periodic bankings are made.

Once again, it cannot be emphasized too strongly that the mixing of sundry cash receipts of this nature, with cash retained for payment of sundry petty cash items, should be discouraged. For payments such as this, a separate cheque should be drawn from the bank periodically, based upon an average weekly or monthly expenditure and replenished from time to time by a cashed cheque drawn on the practice bank account. This should also be kept in a separate cash tin maintained for payment purposes. Doctors and staff requiring cash for any purpose should be asked to complete either a petty cash voucher or to submit a receipt. Once made, all such payments should be regularly and systematically recorded in a petty cash book used only for this purpose. The payments petty cash book should ideally be in the form of an analysis book, which should be regularly added up and balanced and reconciled with the cash held in the tin.

A specimen page from a typical payments petty cash book is shown (Figure 9.1).

Receipts, in the form of cash withdrawn from the bank, should be shown on the left-hand (or debit) side. Payments should be shown on the right-hand (or credit) side, being entered once in the payments (or 'total') column and again in the most appropriate analysis column.

The headings of the various analysis columns depend largely on the circumstances of the particular practice, but again they should be totalled periodically and, if the entries have been made correctly, the sum of the total of the various analysis columns should equal that of the payments (or total column). These can all be totalled monthly and a balance carried forward to the start of the following month. A test balance can be taken at any time, merely by finding the difference between the running totals of the receipts and payments columns. This should then be compared with the cash held in the tin and any difference investigated.

Differences in the cash held may well occur, more often than not for entirely innocent reasons; a payment might have been omitted from the petty cash book or an incorrect entry made. However, the majority of funds passing through the practice will represent payments into and withdrawals from, the practice bank account. We now look at how this should be properly written up and reconciled (see Fig. 9.2).

RECEIPTS		PAYMENTS		Postage		Stationery		Partners' National Insurance		Cleaning		Repairs		Locum fees		Refreshments		Sundries		
32	97																			
		21	95	11	95			10	–											
		5	75			5	75													
		4	50							4	50									
40	–																			
		5	50							5	50									
		1	25															1	25	
		6	80													6	80			
		10	–											10	–					
		4	75									4	75							
		23	60	10	–			13	60											
		2	65			2	65													
		5	25													5	25			
50	–																			
		1	50															1	50	
		4	50															4	50	
		6	50							6	50									
122	97	104	50																	
				21	95	8	40	23	60	16	50	4	75	10	–	12	05	7	25	
		18	47																	
£ 122	97	122	97																	

Figure 9.1: A few days' entries in a typical cash book. A narration giving details of each entry would normally be shown on the left-had side.

Calculating the partners' drawings

In all partnerships there must be a system of withdrawing funds from the practice account by the partners, so that income can be passed to their own accounts for personal use. Doctors, like all other sections of the community, have their personal living expenses to finance and there must be a regular and controlled means of transferring funds to them.

For employees, such as hospital doctors, GP trainees and consultants, this is not a problem. Their salaries will normally be paid to them at the end of each month, having undergone all necessary deductions. GPs, however, are not employees; as we have seen, they are self-employed individuals and, as partners, they have a responsibility to each other. One of these is to ensure that funds passed to them from time to time are in keeping both with their profit-sharing ratios and all other known factors.

The GP's cashbook — recommended column headings.

Receipts

1994	Item	Details	TOTAL	NHS	Appoint-ment	Insurance, Exams etc	Sundry fees	Other receipts
Jan 1	Balance b/forward		2,653 94					2,653 94
	H. Smith – fee	5 –					5 –	
	ABC Insurance Co.	9 –				9 –		
	DEF Insurance Co.	9 –				9 –		
Jan 3	GHI Insurance Co.	9 –				9 –		
	JKL Insurance Co.	9 50				9 50		
	Income tax repaid	127 85						127 85
	County College	350 –			350 –			
Jan 5	MNO Insurance Co.	9 50				9 50		
	Private certificate	2 –					2 –	
Jan 7	B.J. Funeral Crem fee	16 50	547 35				16 50	
Jan 11	PQR Insurance Co.	9 50				9 50		
	STU Insurance Co.	9 –				9 –		
Jan 13	Mr Jones – fee	20 –					20 –	
Jan 14	Mr Brown – fee	25 –					25 –	
	Mr Williams – fee	30 –					30 –	
Jan 17	XYZ Nursing Home	500 –			500 –			
	ABC Insurance Co.	9 50				9 50		
Jan 18	Mr White	20 –					20 –	
Jan 20	Loamshire FHSA	2,350 –	2,350 –	2,350 –				
	GHI Insurance Co.	9 50				9 50		
	Mrs Green	35 –					35 –	
Jan 22	Loamshire Hospital Clinical Assistant	108 96			108 96			
Jan 23	JKL Insurance Co.	9 50				9 50		
Jan 24	Loamshire FHSA	3,647 94	3,647 94	3,647 94				
	Trainee refund	1,000 –						1,000 –
Jan 25	JKL Insurance Co.	9 50				9 50		
	ABC Insurance Co.	9 50				9 50		
	Mr Black	56 –					56 –	
	Mr Blue	25 –					25 –	
Jan 31	Sundry cash takings	55 –					55 –	
	cremation fee	16 50	171 50				16 50	
	Loamshire FHSA Monthly advance	7,250 –	7,250 –	7,250 –				
	Ancillary staff	1,300 –	1,300 –	1,300 –				
		£	18,724 69	14,547 94	958 96	121 –	321 –	3,781 79

Payments

1994	Item	Cheque No.	Sub No.	TOTAL	Salaries	Drugs & instru-ments	Trainee payments	Locum fees	Rent and rates	Lighting & Heating	Cleaning	Tele-phone	Petty Cash	Repairs & rentals	Partners drawings	Tax reserve transfers	Sundries
Jan 1	Dr Jones: locum	635 46	1	100 –				100 –									
	Transfer	S.O.		1,200 –												1,200 –	
Jan 2	Building Society	47	2	85 76													85 76
	Fire Insurance	48	3	2,575 –													2,575 –
Jan 3	Accountancy fees	49	4														
	PAYE/NIC: Month 9			897 40	651 10		246 30										
Jan 4	Smart Drug Company	50	5	35 65		35 65											
	Electricity Board	51	6	152 75						152 75							
	Mrs Jones: cleaner	52		20 –							20 –						
Jan 5	Petty cash	53		50 –									50 –				
	Water Board	54	7	65 35					65 35								
Jan 6	Surgery rent	55	8	1,750 –					1,750 –								
	Gas Board	56	9	97 50						97 50							
Jan 9	Post Office: Telephone	57		267 45								267 45					
Jan 11	Mr Brown: Plumb repair	58		25 –										25 –			
	ZYX Instrument Co.	59		15 50		15 50											
Jan 15	Dr Jones: locum	60		150 –				150 –									
	Cleaning materials	61		27 50							27 50						
Jan 22	Coffee	62		10 75													10 75
Jan 24	Legal charges	63		250 –													250 –
Jan 25	Petty cash	64		50 –									50 –				
Jan 31	Mrs V Williams	65		268 45	268 45												
	Mrs J Smith	66		139 54	139 54												
	Mrs B Jones	67		235 46	235 46												
	Mrs D Johnson	68		226 92	226 92												
	Mrs S Green	69		137 50	137 50												
	Mrs A Watson	70		197 45	197 45												
	Mrs M Robinson	71		226 45	226 45												
	Mrs L White	72		57 50							57 50						
	Dr N Hunt: trainee	73		858 75			858 75										
	Borough Council & rates	S.O.		357 50					357 50								
	Staff pension scheme	S.O.		500 –													500 –
	Dr Grace	S.O.		2,200 –											2,200 –		
	Dr Hobbs	S.O.		2,000 –											2,000 –		
	Dr Bradman	S.O.		1,950 –											1,950 –		
	Dr Hutton	S.O.		675 –											675 –		
				17,856 13													
	Balance c/forward			868 56													
		£		18,724 69	2,082 87	51 15	1,105 05	250 –	2,172 85	250 25	105 –	267 45	100 –	25 –	6,825 –	1,200 –	3,421 51

Figure 9.2: The GP's cashbook – recommended column headings.

Box 9.3: Petty cash recording

Do

Keep the cash proceeds from fees separate from cash used for making payments.

Record cash fee income and pay in to the practice bank account regularly.

Make petty cash payments from float withdrawn from the bank for that purpose.

Record payments in an analysis cash book.

Total columns for each month and balance.

Reconcile balance regularly with cash held in box. Ensure that petty cash drawn from bank is identically shown in both the petty cash receipts and payments cash book.

Do not

Mix up proceeds for cash fees with sundry cash payments.

Keep inadequate records.

Fail to count the cash regularly and check with balance.

Unfortunately, incorrect terminology is often used; it is highly misleading when doctors refer to the monthly amounts paid to them as their 'salary'. This is not the case and the fact cannot be emphasized too strongly. The word 'salary' has all manner of unfortunate connotations in this context, not least being the manner in which the income is taxed, and it is better to avoid the term at all costs.

It is no exaggeration to say that the periodic calculation of partnership drawings is one of the financial procedures which regularly causes most difficulties to GPs in partnership. Many doctors feel that knowledge of their incomes is of such a confidential nature that it cannot be delegated to a member of their staff. These calculations are therefore, in many cases, done by one of the partners themselves. Fortunately, attitudes are changing and, in an increasing number of cases, such drawings calculations are done by a responsible practice manager.

Rather different problems concern the single-handed practitioner. He has no partners to worry about and the money he earns is his own, subject of course to making prudent provisions for income tax and other matters. He may, however, be well advised to pass all his professional transactions through a separate practice bank account and to transfer monthly such sums as can reasonably be set aside into his private bank account for his own use.

Drawings calculations should be done correctly, if partners are to avoid feeling they are receiving more or less than their proper entitlement, and in order to avoid disparities in their current accounts at the end of each financial year.

Whether drawings have been properly calculated or not will become evident when the annual partnership accounts are prepared; any differences between the current accounts of the partners will then become apparent. Steps should be taken to see that such errors do not recur and that the balances are adjusted by subsequent and 'one-off' adjustments to drawings.

There are probably as many different systems of drawings by partners as there are fingers on one's hands. Whatever system is used, it is essential that it is operated properly. The simplest system would apply in a two-man partnership sharing profits equally, so that both doctors could withdraw identical amounts. In practice, that is likely to be the exception rather than the rule. In virtually all cases, complex adjustments will be made for differing rates of seniority awards; superannuation payments; added years contributions; loan interest charges; national insurance; repayments of leave advance, and other items.

The system which is perhaps most widely used in partnerships is the 'month-end' or 'quarter-end' system, under which partners are paid out at the end of each month, and adjustments made quarterly to take into consideration the factors mentioned above. Whilst it is acceptable that payments at the end of the two intermediate months may be made in partnership ratios, the full measure of adjustments must be made at the end of the quarter. This is illustrated by the example shown in Figure 9.3. This shows a four-doctor partnership, Drs A, B, C and D, the three senior partners having a share of 28% and a new partner, Dr D, with a share of 16%. Drs A and B are both paying for added years (A); all the partners are paying leave advances (B); whilst Dr D has a loan from the GP Finance Corporation (C). Drs A, B, C and D have seniority awards at varying rates (D). The figures shown are for illustration purposes only and it should not be assumed that these will apply to partnerships in practice.

In computing the total amount to be distributed, it is normal to find the balance available on the partnership bank account (F), either by reference to the bank statements at the end of the quarter or, more preferably and where adequate and accurate records are kept, by referring to the balance in hand as shown in the practice cash book. There should be retained from the amount the estimated expenditure to run the practice during the succeeding months (G), and the balance will then be available for distribution (H).

It should be remembered that, at the same time as this distribution is made, certain deductions have been made from the quarterly FHSA remuneration and, similarly, certain additions will have been included (see Box 9.4). It is necessary to reverse these entries before arriving at the total allocation for the quarter and then to allocate the proper amounts to each of the four partners.

It may also be that certain of the partners do not own the surgery premises and they will not be entitled to share in any notional rent allowances in respect of the building. A detailed examination of the quarterly FHSA statement should be made, in order to ensure that all items of this nature are taken into account. Care should also be taken to see that all the income to be distributed has been earned during a period when current profit-sharing ratios were in operation. In many cases, NHS income is paid substantially in arrears. It should ideally be allocated to the period in which it was actually earned and, where such items of income have been received during one quarter, these should be taken out of the normal quarterly calculation and divided separately, in appropriate ratios.

Equalized drawings systems

Many partnerships are now becoming aware of systems of equalized drawings, under which a full year's net income is estimated and divided into equal amounts for distribution to the partners. Provided that all proper adjustments have been made, this regular monthly withdrawal can be paid to the partners' personal bank accounts by standing order.

This system allows a partner to estimate his regular monthly income, for the purpose of his personal family budget, and also avoids the constant calculation and issue of monthly cheques. The system is illustrated in Figure 9.4, for a four-doctor partnership with varying rates of superannuation, seniority, added years and other items. This calculation is normally made on a tax year basis, so that a reserve can be made for the annual partnership income tax liability.

Box 9.4: Details of likely items to be adjusted on periodic drawings calculations

Income
- Seniority awards.
- Postgraduate education allowances.
- Notional rent allowances (where to be distributed in different ratios to partnership shares).

Outgoings
- Superannuation contributions: standard.
- Added years and unreduced lump sum.
- National Insurance contributions.
- Repayment of leave advances.
- GPFC (or other loan repayments and interest).
- Transfers to income tax reserve.

Drs, A, B, C and D	Total £	Dr A 28%	Dr B 28%	Dr C 28%	Dr D 16%
Balance in partnership bank account (F)	13 000				
Less:					
retain on hand (G)	4500				
For distribution (H)		8500			
Add deductions:					
Superannuation	540				
Added years (A)	120				
Leave advance (B)	1200				
GPFC loan (C)	125				
Monthly on account	10 000	11 985			
		20 485			
Less additional income:					
Seniority (D)		2800			
For allocation (in partnership ratios)		17 685	4952	4952	4952	2829
Add:					
Seniority (D)		2800	1000	1000	400	400
		20 485	5952	5952	5352	3229
Less:					
Superannuation	540		150	150	150	90
Added years (A)	120		75	45		300
Leave advance (B)	1200		300	300	300	125
GPFC loan (C)	125	1985	— 525	495	450	515
		18 500	5427	5457	4902	2714
Less: paid monthly on account		10 000	2800	2800	2800	1600
Net withdrawals		8500	2627	2657	2102	1114

Figure 9.3: Calculation of quarterly drawings, October 1993.

The detailed preparation of such an equalized drawings system will normally be done by the partnership accountant, who should have the required detailed information available to him, and who will be in a position to calculate the tax reserve to be operated during any given period.

The use of income tax reserve accounts

We have had a look at the manner in which drawings calculations are made and that these must take into account the practice's tax liabilities. Tax is normally payable in two instalments on 1 January and 1 July. Many practices, for reasons of cash flow benefit and security, prefer to set regular amounts

	Total	Dr A (28%) £	Dr B (28%) £	Dr C (24%) £	Dr D (20%) £
Estimated partnership profits for year	90 000	25 200	25 200	21 600	18 000
Seniority awards	7400	3900	2000	—	1500
Total income (est) (1)	97 400	29 100	27 200	21 600	19 500
Deductions					
Superannuation (est)	5600	1600	1500	1300	1200
Added years	1300	800	300	200	—
Outside appts (est)	100	—	20	80	—
National insurance (est)					
Class I (appointments)	100	—	—	100	—
Class II (stamps)	960	240	240	240	240
Repayment of leave advance	4824	1206	1206	1206	1206
Repayment of loans (GPFC)	1300	—	—	500	800
	14 184	3846	3266	3626	3446
Income tax reserve transfers	18 000	6500	5500	4000	2000
Total outgoings (2)	32 184	10 346	8766	7626	5446
Net (1–2)	65 216	18 754	18 434	13 974	14 054
Monthly	5434	1563	1536	1164	1171
(rounded down)	5415	1560	1530	1160	1165

Figure 9.4: Calculation of equalized drawings for the year to June 1994.

aside in a separate deposit or building society account, from which these payments might be made as and when they fall due. Systems of this nature have two main advantages.

1 They avoid the drawing of large cheques by individual partners twice a year, often with fairly traumatic effects on the individual's own finances.
2 They avoid the possibility of a retiring partner leaving a tax liability behind him, which may fall on the continuing partners.

The timescale for the operation of such a reserve is important and to a great degree depends on the estimates of future liabilities being received as early as possible within each separate tax year.

Under the normal preceding year basis of assessment, a practice with a year-end on, say 30 June, will find that the profits earned in the year ending on that date will be assessable in the following tax year. In the case of a practice making up its accounts to 30 June 1993, the tax assessment based on those profits would be for the tax year 1994/95. It would normally be possible for an accountant to make a reasonable estimate of the tax payable before the start of the actual year of assessment. With a 31 March year-end, however, it may be May or June before even a preliminary estimate can be prepared.

	Annual tax liability 1994/95 £	Monthly reserve April 1994–March 1995 £
Dr W	6000	495
Dr X	5000	410
Dr Y	4750	390
Dr Z	2250	185
	18 000	1480

The monthly transfer can be slightly less than 1/12 of the annual liability, due to interest which will be credited to the account.

Figure 9.5:   Income tax reserve.

The reserve should be held physically separate from the main partnership funds, either in a building society or bank deposit account, and the periodic interest divided between the partners in proportion to their shares of the balance on hand. It should preferably be transferred by means of a monthly standing order from the main partnership bank account, on a tax year basis so that for, say, the 1994/95 year, 12 monthly transfers would be made, from the end of April 1994 until March 1995.

A typical reserve is illustrated in Figure 9.5, which shows a four-doctor practice with an estimated liability for 1994/95 of £18 000. This could have been calculated in January or February 1994. Interest will be credited to the various partners in proportions to their different contributions.

Surgery premises

One other aspect in which the finance of medical practices is significantly different from that of other businesses is that concerning the means by which surgery premises are financed.

Basically, for doctors practising from surgeries predominantly for the use of NHS patients, either a refund of rental payments is made, in the case of doctors practising from rented surgeries or, in the case of surgeries owned by the partners an allowance, in the form of either a notional or cost-rent allowance, will be paid to the practice.

Rented surgeries

These may fall under a number of different headings. Firstly, a fairly basic case of a surgery rented from a third-party landlord, to whom a rent is paid. It will be necessary for the rent receipt to be submitted to the FHSA after payment and this should be done as soon as possible. Provided that the whole of the surgery or building subject to the rent charge is allowable and falls under the qualifying rules, a full refund will be made.

Health centres

Many doctors practice from health centres and should ensure that the charge for rent and rates, which will not actually pass through the accounts of the practice, is ascertained. This should be handed to the accountant as he will be required to show it in the annual accounts as an item of expense and refund each year.

Proportions of ownership

It may well be that the surgery is owned by not all the partners in the practice and indeed arrangements of this nature are extremely common, probably because some or all of the partners who may not have a full-time commitment, do not wish to become involved in property ownership.

It is important that this is established as it affects the allocation of the rent allowance and the cost of servicing any loans which have been taken out to buy or develop the property. It is important that this is understood, is shown clearly in the partnership deed and, if necessary, reflected in the drawings calculations.

Cost-rent schemes

Schemes of developing new, or adapting additional, surgery buildings under the cost-rent scheme are now extremely common and are an excellent means by which the partners in a practice can acquire a valuable interest in a commercial building without any appreciable capital outlay.

Such schemes are extremely complex both in their initial organization and in their subsequent administration. This should not be embarked upon without lengthy detailed and knowledgeable advice from professional people: an architect, a solicitor and an accountant, experienced in this type of work. This should be done in partnership with your FHSA who has the last word in deciding what the rent allowance will be and the means by which it will be calculated. (See *Making Sense of the Cost Rent Scheme*, Radcliffe Medical Press.)

The role of the accountant

The average practice will use many financial advisers during its normal operations. Some of these, such as the lawyer and the architect they may well see infrequently, the bank manager probably at rather more frequent intervals. But it will be the accountant who effectively will have overall control over the practice finances, to whom they will most closely relate and who will be in most ready contact with them. In practice this contact is likely to take place via the practice manager, who will be responsible for reporting to her doctors the recommendations of the accountant on numerous matters, including drawings, tax reserves, etc.

It is very important that the accountant should be one who has specialized in medical finance, hopefully for many years and has a umber of GP clients from whom he can gather his experience and speciality. Many practices find difficulty in relating to an accountant who does not understand the strange ways of doctors' finances and express constant dissatisfaction.

The relationship between the doctor, the practice manager and the accountant should properly be one of confidence and even friendship.

All too often and unfortunately it degenerates, possibly through misunderstandings on both sides, to mutual resentment and often to a parting of the ways. Many practices, through lack of knowledge of the accountant's function, find it difficult to judge whether he is doing his job properly and this guideline could well assist in consolidating their views. In judging potential candidates for the practice accountant, a number of criteria should be borne in mind.

Is he a specialist?

Does he have a copy of the Red Book and is he conversant with topics of medical finance, such as cost-rent schemes, doctors superannuation, practice allowances and numerous other items?

Efficiency

Are letters answered promptly and telephone calls returned? Are the accounts delivered within a relatively brief period; are tax, pension queries, etc. dealt with expeditiously?

Fee levels

This is discussed in more detail below but generally speaking the level of fees charged should not be a major item in deciding who will be the practice accountant. Of far more importance is whether he is capable, and demonstrates his ability to do an efficient and specialist job for the practice.

Proximity

Many practices feel they need an accountant working virtually from the next street. With modern methods of communication this is by no means as necessary as it might have been in the past. The times when the practice manager or doctors will need to consult their accountant personally in the same office will usually be few and far between and most accountants will arrange in any event to visit the practice at least once or twice yearly for a full discussion.

Fees

All accountants calculate their fees by means of an hourly charge which may vary from firm to firm but which will reflect the seniority, experience and aptitude of the individual partner or staff member dealing with the work.

It follows that it is in the interest of the practice to minimize that work so much as is possible. For instance, a bookkeeping system on the lines illustrated on page 170 will almost certainly result in a lower level of fees than a system which is either non-existent, inadequately written up or inaccurately presented. Accountants' fees will include an addition of 17.5% VAT, which is not part of the actual fee retained by the accountant but must be paid over by him to the Inland Revenue. Nevertheless, as doctors are unable to register for VAT it is effectively an additional cost to their practice.

The judgement of accounting fees is extremely difficult and dependent on numerous factors, but as a very rough and general guideline, fee levels, which exclude personal work for the individual partners, should probably fall within the range of 0.5% to 1% of gross practice income. If they exceed that level, the practice will be quite reasonable in expecting justification to be supplied. On the other hand, if these fall below those factors, there could be a possibility that the accountant is spending insufficient time on the practice affairs, or using inexperienced staff. A practice with a gross turnover, including fee income and refunds, of £800 000 could probably expect therefore an annual charge, at current fee levels, in the order of £4000 inclusive of VAT, but exclusive of work done on the partners' personal affairs.

Duties

The accountant's duties will be many and varied. Basically he will prepare the practice accounts, having these agreed both by the partners and by the Inland Revenue for tax purposes. In addition he should be prepared to give additional advice on such matters as surgery development; calculation of tax reserves and drawings; provide statistical and management information concerning the practice income, expenditure and profits; advise the doctors on their pension arrangements; deal with personal tax affairs, claiming of practice expenses and numerous other items. It follows that he should be familiar with the Red Book and be able to interpret this as required.

Upon engagement an accountant should always be asked to give a quotation of his fees and should be expected to stick by this unless there are any factors of which he was not aware at the time it was made.

The role of the practice manager

It is no exaggeration to say that a qualified, experienced and committed practice manager is probably the most important person in the efficiently run practice. She (or increasingly he) should be the equivalent of a company secretary, with control over the finances, administration, management and staffing of the practice below partner level. She should attend and participate in practice meetings and generally act as guide, philosopher and friend to her doctors.

The emphasis in the job title is on the work 'manager': the practice 'manager' should be the head of the team. Yet, in some practices the practice manager is not taken into the confidence of the doctors, and is thus excluded from the ultimate management function. She is treated as little more than a superior receptionist/secretary and has little part to play in the decision-making processes. This is ultimately to the detriment of the practice.

One of the more important tasks of the practice manager is the control of the practice finances; to ensure that these are run in an efficient and systematic manner, to maximize the practice income, keep a control on expenditure and hence increase the profitability of the practice.

Good management involves successful delegation of responsibility and the manager in general practice must be prepared, where necessary, to ensure that part of her workload is delegated to more junior staff, whom it will be more cost-effective to employ for that purpose.

Many practices fall into the trap of not adequately defining the practice manager's role; she may lack a full job description – or even, in some cases, a contract of employment – and may find herself taking conflicting instructions from different partners. She will therefore feel unappreciated and unfulfilled.

At the other end of the scale, a few enlightened practices have sought to give practical recognition of the importance of the practice manager's role by elevating her to partner status. Such a step, whilst generally to be welcomed, can create problems with regard to her taxation position, with liability in professional negligence cases, and in relations with other senior staff.

10 Fundholding

Background

The concept of fundholding is the latest, and perhaps the most far reaching, change in the delivery of patient care since the NHS was conceived. It was outlined in a White Paper *Working for Patients* published in 1989. This document gave the plans for the future of the NHS and the main initiative was the introduction of general practice fundholding. In 1990 the GP Contract was introduced, which shifted the emphasis away from basic allowances to a greater number of item of service payments and increased capitation fees. In other words, to maintain a level of income each GP needed to provide a full range of patient services. Almost by default, each practice had to become more businesslike in its approach to utilizing resources, or suffer the consequence of a drop in income. General practitioners were ideally placed to spearhead a major initiative to identify and improve the services needed by their patients. They were also the best equipped in terms of business experience, most practices having a defined management structure, decision-making forum and an in-built accountability to colleagues and patients.

There are many arguments for and against fundholding, both political and ethical, however this chapter will ignore these debates and deal with the current parameters of the scheme.

Who's who in fundholding

These are the major players in the fundholding system:

Secretary of State	The Cabinet Minister responsible for the National Health Service.
NHSME	National Health Service Management Executive – responsible for policy decisions.
RHA	Regional Health Authority – responsible for interpreting the NHSME's decisions

	and communicating them to FHSAs and GP fundholders. Arbiters in the event of disagreements between FHSAs and GP fundholders about budget setting or fundholding policies.
FHSA	Family Heath Services Authority – responsible for liaison with GP fundholders, monitoring, budget setting negotiations, training, and routine queries.
GPFH	General Practice Fundholders – those practices who have successfully completed a preparatory year and who have been allocated a budget.
Providers	Hospitals or Units which provide patient services following a referral from a GP.

The scope of the budget

Funding is allocated under four headings:

1 staff salaries
2 drugs and appliances
3 hospital services
4 community nursing.

Each portion of the budget is inter-changeable, i.e. the overall position of the fund at the end of each financial year is the net result of the total budget, not individual elements.

At the moment, the budget-setting process is largely based upon historical expenditure. However, over the next few years, there will be a swing towards capitation based funding. There are many factors which affect a capitation formulae and one of the difficulties in the introduction of such a system has been the absence of a method that is universally acceptable. Each practice perceives that they have special needs that should be reflected in their budget. This has to be balanced against a health service that is cash limited and which must be seen to be fair to all parties in the allocation of funds.

There are some pilot studies that bring other responsibilities under the jurisdiction of the GP fundholder, and these are outlined at the end of this chapter.

The preparatory year

To be offered a budget, each practice must complete a preparatory year to demonstrate that suitable levels of expertise and technology are available to manage the fund, to train the doctors and staff, and to identify the monitoring systems and data collection necessary to track performance and negotiate an adequate budget.

Priorities for the preparatory year

Identify the person/people responsible for the management of the budget

There are several options to consider when deciding who will take responsibility for fund management on behalf of the practice, all of which will require some alteration to the personnel structure of the practice. When planning this aspect, the most important considerations are the skills required, not the person. Fundholding has tremendous implications on all areas of the practice and it should not be judged in isolation. Good communication skills are vital, whether it is to persuade secretaries to take copies of all referral letters and replies, to explain to doctors the effect of their personal referral patterns on the budget or to ask nurses to keep records of all the specimens they send to the laboratories. These skills must also be evident when dealing with outside bodies such as the FHSA, RHA, hospital contracts, the business manager, other fundholding colleagues or auditors. Most of the technical skills can be learned, for example, using the fundholding software, completing returns for the FHSA and RHA, monitoring activity and checking invoices. However, a genuine interest in fundholding and patient care must be present if the individual is to gain any form of job satisfaction. Without that particular motivation fundholding would become mundane and lack the flair that results in so many innovations.

Management options
1 **Fundholding partner.** This has the advantage of bringing clinical expertise to fund management, but the time involved may result in an unequal patient workload. This in turn could become a bone of contention within the partnership, especially as there is no statutory provision to employ a locum for more than one half day per week.
2 **Existing practice manager.** If the existing practice manager has appropriate skills and an interest in fundholding there is no reason why he or she should not perform a dual role. This cannot be done without additional support in the shape of a deputy or similar to free sufficient time. Practice management and fund management are full time roles and it

Box 10.1: Fund manager job description

Budget setting
- To provide all relevant information to verify budget offers.
- To liaise with FHSA or RHA in the event of a difference between activity and budget offer.

Monitoring
- To enter all relevant patient contacts that are part of fundholding into the computer software.
- To follow all RHA and FHSA guidelines when entering data.
- To produce timely end of month reports.
- To complete statutory monitoring forms.
- To check performance against anticipated levels and advise the partners of any areas of concern.
- To train the staff involved in data collection and data entry on the fundholding software.

Contracting
- To attend all meetings with hospital business managers of major providers.
- To be a positive part of the negotiating process.
- To make necessary information available to other members of the practice team if they are involved in any contract negotiations.
- To monitor levels of activity and quality standards as specified in current contracts.
- To undertake regular patient surveys to assess quality standards from a consumer's point of view.
- to obtain the best possible financial and quality package to reflect the services required to meet patients' needs.

Management
- To be involved in formulating policies to accommodate fundholding.
- To create and audit all systems to support fundholding.
- To advise partners of the budget status on a monthly basis.
- To take an active part in local consortium groups.
- To facilitate audit meetings, eg rationalizing prescribing and practice formulary, that have a direct impact on fundholding.

Box 10.1: *continued*

- To check each invoice in detail and liaise with providers in the event of discrepancies.
- To maintain effective communication channels between the practice and consultants, business managers; other fundholding and non-fundholding practices.
- To facilitate fundholding protocols, eg preferred consultants and providers.
- To research and present potential innovations for discussion with the partners.

---

would be unrealistic to expect one person to accommodate the latter within their normal working week without delegating the routine aspects of running the practice.
3 **Fund manager.** There may be a person within the organization willing to become responsible for the budget. This would be an advantage, especially when assessing the impact of certain fundholding tasks on the rest of the practice and if that person was able to cope with the transition from 'team member' to 'manager'. Many practices have opted to recruit a fund manager from the commercial world, and business acumen can be beneficial in a fundholding environment.
4 **Fundholding partner and practice manager.** This may seem like the course of least resistance but the dual responsibility does combat the feeling of isolation in fund management and combines clinical and management skills very effectively. Many partnerships operate an 'executive partner' system to liaise with the practice manager on various aspects of practice management, and this becomes an extension of that system. It has the added advantage of flexibility when it comes to attending meetings, and cover when one person is absent.

Each practice functions differently and there is no correct answer when it comes to appointing a fund manager. The right course of action is the one that brings the correct range of skills and accountability to running the fund.

Monitor staff salaries

The budget is intended to reimburse 70% of gross staff salaries plus 100% of the employer's National Insurance contributions for recognized categories of practice staff. The practice must be able to prove a minimum contribution of at least 30% to gross staff salaries from partnership funds. This is the element of the budget that is completely under the control of the practice, the easiest to monitor and to assess the sums needed to staff the practice efficiently. All practices have some kind of salaries ledger, either a manual or computer system, and are already familiar with providing end of year returns to the Inland Revenue and the practice accountant. This information base can be analysed to become a management tool for the staff budget.

It will be necessary to break down the gross salaries into the components, ie:

- basic salary
- additional cover for sickness
- additional cover for holidays
- training.

By doing this a pattern will emerge, and some elements will be on-going whilst others will be 'one-offs'. The on-going items are likely to be the cover required for holidays (because it is possible to calculate the amount of holiday time that will need cover), and the likely spread throughout the year. The 'one-offs' will be things like compassionate leave, long-term sickness absence and special practice projects that have required additional staffing. These need not be included in longer term planning as they are not likely to recur.

This example shows how rapidly a basic staffing level of 1300 hours per month can increase by 10.06% when all the other factors are added into the planning. This could be the difference between an adequate staffing budget and insufficient funding.

Some practices may have to look seriously at transferring funds from other elements of the budget when a capitation formula is introduced, or making

---

Box 10.2: Analysis of salaries (in hours, based on 12 staff working 25 hours per week each)

	Basic hours	Holiday cover	Sickness cover	Training	Other	Total
April	1300	75	10	8	0	1393
May	1300	25	0	0	10	1335
June	1300	50	0	8	10	1368
July	1300	150	20	0	0	1470
August	1300	350	25	0	0	1675
September	1300	225	25	0	0	1550
October	1300	175	25	16	20	1536
November	1300	0	0	16	20	1336
December	1300	0	50	0	0	1350
January	1300	25	50	0	0	1375
February	1300	50	15	16	10	1391
March	1300	75	0	16	0	1391
	15 600	1200	220	80	70	17 170

up the difference from practice profits. Many FHSAs are including general practitioners and practice managers in working parties to devise capitation formulae and such elements as ethnicity, branch surgeries, areas of deprivation and local morbidity are under consideration.

Monitor expenditure on drugs and appliances

The Prescription Pricing Authority produces monthly statements outlining the expenditure on drugs and appliances each month, a full explanation of the levels of PACT data is given in Chapter 12.

These statements should be reviewed monthly, and any trends or areas picked up where prescribing could be rationalized or a greater use made of generic drugs. A working party that includes all partners and any nurses running chronic disease clinics needs to be established early in the preparatory year. The secret to successfully controlling prescribing is a practice formulary that is 'owned' by all the clinicians. Without such ownership it will be ignored and valuable hours wasted. Established prescribing methods cannot be changed over-night and regular discussions can help to highlight new information and facilitate change in a non-threatening way.

Monitor the activity for hospital services

This is the most difficult area to monitor because of the variety of specialties and providers that have been traditionally used for patient referrals. It is essential that these are all identified and quantified during the preparatory year. Without such information a budget offer cannot be verified or negotiated. It is not enough to say 'we think we have . . .', and budgets can only be amended if accurate evidence is produced. It is not a new concept to monitor referrals – every practice should be collating such data for the annual practice report. Fundholding simply demands greater detail and includes the number of follow-ups in out-patient clinics, type and number of in-patient episodes and day cases.

It is essential that all activity is recorded, and to do this effectively usually requires a means to intercept all practice mail. Each practice will devise its own system, but whatever the method the important message is 'collect everything'. Additional copies can be taken of all referral letters originated by the practice, all in-coming referral replies, discharge summaries and investigation results need to be either copied or recorded daily. The system needs to be 100% accurate, as partial data is meaningless when verifying a budget offer in the future.

Hints:

- a weekly data collection sheet for doctors to tick in surgery each time they instigate an investigation, X-ray or physiotherapy referral

- train all secretaries to give an additional copy of every referral letter written to the fund manager
- have all mail delivered to a central point for opening and sorting
- devise a method for dealing with mail that arrives on Saturdays
- apply a clinical code to all in-patient episodes to allow effective price banding to compare with budget offer
- ask yourself 'can I tell if each element of the budget offer is reasonable?'
- obtain the waiting lists from each hospital to verify and cost them
- liaise with community nursing staff to gather information about any referral they may make to a chargeable service, eg speech therapy.

Training

The importance of training the whole team cannot be stressed strongly enough. To incorporate new systems to capture activity information will require some adjustment of attitudes and existing procedures. Each item needs to be thought through carefully and discussed with the whole practice team.

The FHSA or RHA will hold training seminars and workshops during the preparatory year to help practices to identify their fundholding objectives and to facilitate appropriate data collection. It is an advantage if more than one person can attend such training meetings, not just for moral support but also to guard against unexpected resignations or sickness. For this reason, the fund management structure including the data entry staff and responsible GP, needs to be organized at the start of the preparatory year.

Prepare a practice business plan

Some practices may find the information that they are required to provide to become fundholders intrusive. However, a fundholding budget is in the public domain and, as such, subject to public scrutiny. Any prospective fundholding practice must be prepared to be accountable for all of their actions to the FHSA, RHA, auditors, colleagues, Community Health Council and patients.

The practice will be expected to complete a comprehensive application form to become fundholders, which includes an outline business plan. This should incorporate a description of the practice premises, the personnel planned to manage the budget, current patient services, a description of the practice population, and any external factors that may necessitate future changes. From this base line the practice can identify the way in which it wishes to progress and compare current services available and match them to the needs of the patients. The final part is to outline the steps that the practice will take to introduce or improve any services with the yardsticks that will be used to monitor their success.

Box 10.3: Business Plan

1 Evaluation of current situation:
   - staffing levels
   - premises
   - practice population
   - management and decision making structure
   - skills.
2 Set practice aims and objectives:
   - mission statement
   - overall plans for the future
   - match current services against patient needs
   - identify areas that require improvement.
3 Devise action plans:
   - tasks to be performed
   - individual responsibilities for those tasks
   - timescales
   - elements to be audited.
4 Measure achievement against aims and objectives.

Which computer software system?

There are several companies who have passed the Department of Health conformance testing for fundholding software, and the practice must decide which one is compatible with their existing system and fulfil their fundholding needs. There are several sources from which to obtain advice – the FHSA, the RHA, the existing computer maintenance company and the GP system company. Time should be taken to review carefully each option available and place an order several months before the new financial year. Staff will need to be trained and be given enough time to become familiar with the chosen system before fundholding begins for real.

Always make a final check with the FHSA that the computer software that you have chosen has passed all the necessary conformance tests.

Establish professional links

Fundholding can be a frightening thought, especially during the preparatory year. The fund manager may also feel quite isolated as there is no-one else in the practice directly comparable, or subject to the same demands. It is helpful to find out the names of all the other local fundholders and make contact with their managers. Not everyone will belong to the same wave, but there will be someone who has recently completed the preparatory year who can identify closely with any concerns. However, it is not fair to expect another practice to train you for free. The management allowance exists for just such expenses and training is a legitimate way of using these monies effectively. Apart from other practices, there are often local meetings, or help can be obtained from the National Association of Fundholding Practices, the FHSA and the RHA. Start attending meetings to identify sources of information as soon as possible.

The management allowance

The management allowance exists for practices to use to offset certain expenses that have been necessary as a direct result of fundholding. The allowance for the preparatory year 1993/94 is £17 500 and the FHSA will require a plan of expenditure at the beginning of the year. This increases to £35 000 when the practice has accepted a budget and progresses to full fundholding.

Acceptable expenditure
- 100% of staff costs for fundholding duties, eg data entry, data collection and contract negotiation.
- The employment of a locum (subject to a maximum) for one half day per week to allow a partner to do fundholding duties.
- Office costs for fundholding data, eg copying and postage.
- A limited amount for small capital items, eg fax machine.
- Staff costs for fundholding training.
- Improvements to premises, but only after approval by the RHA and FHSA.
- Rent of additional office space for fundholding.

The management allowance is held by the FHSA and they will require evidence of how the money has been spent before reimbursing the practice. It is sensible to devise a claim form (*see* Fig. 10.1) to keep accurate monthly records and open a bank account exclusively for this money. This will avoid any complications between practice and fundholding accounts and allow the management allowance to be tracked easily by the FHSA, auditors and speed up the completion of any official returns.

Accepting a budget

The budget offer comes in a series of 'cuts', known as first cut, second cut and so on. It is also broken down into the four elements of staff budget, drug budget, hospital services budget and community nursing budget.

```
┌─────────────────────────────────────────────────────────────┐
│  Management allowance claim form 1993/94                       │
│                                                                │
│                                                                │
│  Dr Smith & Partners                                           │
│  1, High Street,                                               │
│  Anytown                                                       │
│                                                                │
│                                                                │
│  Month: ─────────────────────────────                         │
│                                                                │
│                                   ┌──────────────────────┐    │
│  Items claimed:                   │      Amount:          │    │
│                                   ├──────────────────────┤    │
│                                   │                      │    │
│                                   ├──────────────────────┤    │
│                                   │                      │    │
│                                   ├──────────────────────┤    │
│                                   │                      │    │
│                                   ├──────────────────────┤    │
│                                   │                      │    │
│                                   ├──────────────────────┤    │
│                                   │                      │    │
│                         Total     ├──────────────────────┤    │
│                                   │                      │    │
│  Special notes:                   └──────────────────────┘    │
│                                                                │
└─────────────────────────────────────────────────────────────┘
```

Figure 10.1:   Sample management allowance claim form.

When each cut arrives it must be given priority and, after appropriate analysis, comments returned to the FHSA, with any supporting evidence.

Staff salaries

As explained earlier in the chapter, the budget is currently based on current expenditure and a percentage of a capitation based calculation. When reviewing the budget offer it should be remembered that 100% of fundholding staff salaries can be taken from the management allowance, and this portion should be identified and deducted from the remaining staff salaries. The same criteria apply for reimbursement (as in the Red Book), in other words, only recognized categories of staff are eligible. Fundholding will not allow for gardeners or cleaners to be taken from the staffing budget!

The budget is paid to the practice in twelfths at the end of each month. Again, it is essential to have a separate staff salaries account for this money to be paid into and the practice must be able to demonstrate that at least 30% has been paid from the partnership account. The FHSA may be willing to pay the staff budget a few days ahead of the month end to assist the practice's cash flow, but this requires discussion and their approval.

The FHSA will need a quarterly return to be completed which identifies gross salaries, employer's National Insurance, relief hours and any salaries taken from the management allowance.

It will be easier in the long-term if accurate monthly records and a monthly reconciliation with the salary bank account are done. This will make the quarterly returns and end of year reconciliations quicker and more accurate (*see* Fig. 10.2).

Staff salaries		Dr Smith & Partners 1, High Street Anytown
Month: _____		
	Gross salaries	Employer's N.I.
From salaries ledger DEDUCT Salaries from management allowance	_____ _____	_____ _____
NET COSTS	(a) _____	(b) _____
Salaries from budget = Net Gross salaries × 70% plus employer's N.I.	(a) × 70%	(c) _____ (b) _____
=	(d) _____	
Monthly budget less Actual salaries Over/under spend	(e) _____ (d) _____ (e)–(d) _____	

Figure 10.2:   Sample salary calculation.

This information needs to be entered into the fundholding software each month to calculate the month end statements. These statements must be reconciled to the cash in the salaries account.

Drug budget

For the management of the prescribing budget please refer to Chapter 12.

The fund manager needs to ensure that a copy of the monthly PACT statements sent to each partner reach the fundholding office. The information is then entered into the fundholding software to calculate the month end statements. The drug expenditure from the fundholding software should equal the amount shown on the PACT statements.

Hospital services

Every fundholding patient contact must be entered into the fundholding software, and to do this the databases must be complete (*see* Fig. 10.3). At

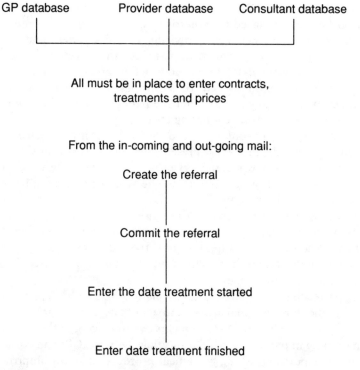

Figure 10.3:   Data flow for each episode of care.

the beginning of each financial year the practice must enter the providers, consultants, contracts, treatments and prices into the software. The list of fundholding procedures, ie the clinical codings, are written into the software specification.

There is a facility on the software to cancel referrals if the treatment start date has not been entered. There is also a facility to unpick a referral between treatment started and treatment finished. This may vary from one version of the software to another and these points should be covered during initial training or in the explanatory notes that accompany each upgrade.

The practice data entry forms part of a greater cycle to monitor activity and expenditure, and should be directly matched to the provider's information (see Fig. 10.4).

When providers send an invoice it must be verified in accordance with the contract and the patient's attendance checked. For example, if the contract states that there will be a consultant's letter after each out-patient appointment then this must be in the patient's notes before payment is authorized. It is fair to say that communications from hospitals have improved considerably since fundholding began, and GPs have an opportunity to intercept patient care if it is inappropriate. This could apply to high re-attendance specialties, like rheumatology. It must, of course, be an agreement between the consultant and the GP.

The GP is ideally placed to monitor hospital services on purely clinical grounds, as they have personal knowledge of every patient and can track individuals through the system. Waiting times can be accurately monitored and areas of concern tackled by the contracting process. Ultimately, fundholders have the option to take their business elsewhere if a particular department or hospital does not offer the patient care the GP would wish, and this can be a powerful negotiating tool.

Providers will have to conform to a '6 week rule' for invoicing from 1 April 1994. In other words, they must present their invoices within six weeks of the end of the month in which the service was performed. The exception will be if the invoice was originally sent to the wrong practice and has to be re-processed to the correct one.

The onus is on each practice to devise in-house monitoring procedures to identify problem areas, eg long waiting times, and then to be seen to deal with them. The contract is a mixture of activity data and quality standards and both are important if the practice is to secure high standards of care and achieve good value for money.

It is up to each practice to forge good relationships with hospital contracts managers and business managers, and maintain open channels of communication to expedite any disagreements over invoicing. If there is a clinical forum running in parallel, ie regular meetings between GPs and consultants, there is an opportunity to agree clinical protocols that will improve care, discourage inappropriate referrals and be cost effective for both providers

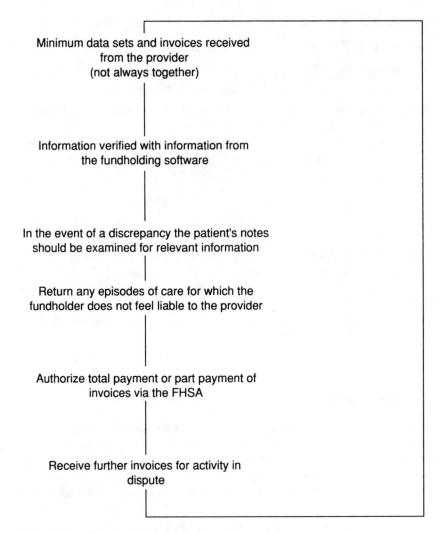

Minimum data sets and invoices received
from the provider
(not always together)

Information verified with information from
the fundholding software

In the event of a discrepancy the patient's notes
should be examined for relevant information

Return any episodes of care for which the
fundholder does not feel liable to the provider

Authorize total payment or part payment of
invoices via the FHSA

Receive further invoices for activity in
dispute

Figure 10.4: Data flow for invoices.

and GP fundholders. In the event of a total disagreement, the FHSA and RHA
will act as arbiters to interpret the standard guidelines.

The contracting process

Types of contracts

Block: An agreed sum of money for all activity, ie no floor or
                          ceiling for activity.

Cost and volume: An agreed sum of money for a specified level of activity.

Cost per case: Each patient episode is charged separately.

Non-attributable: Introduced to deal with contracts where the budget is
                      'blocked back', eg community nursing.

These types of contracts are those usually used by major providers; however, there are also a range of hospitals used only occasionally for specific services. The whole point of fundholding is freedom of referral and 'one-offs' (often away from the immediate area) where a contract does not exist to allow practices to make extra contractual referrals. These are always on a cost per case basis.

The first step in the contracting process starts within the practice. The partners need to be aware of their historical referral patterns and pool their views on the levels of service received. From this a desirable range of contracts to be placed will emerge, and the fund manager and/or executive partner will take this information to the various contracting meetings. The creation of a 'preferred consultants' list will have other benefits to the practice and will be helpful to new partners and GP trainees. To remain effective it must be updated annually to include new consultants and remove those who retire or whose performance is deemed to be lacking.

Moving contracts to alternative providers

One of the main advantages of being a fundholding practice is the ability to place contracts with a chosen provider. If every fundholder had total freedom with their budget it could have disastrous results for certain providers and over-load others. For this reason, the amount of flexibility is limited for the initial years of fundholding to prevent destabilization of traditional referral patterns.

Year 1   20% flexibility in hospital services budget
          80% traditional referral patterns

Year 2   40% flexibility in hospital services budget
          60% traditional referral patterns

Year 3   100% freedom to place hospital services budget with any provider.

In September or October the FHSA will ask each fundholding practice for an indication of any major shifts they may make for the following financial year. These include a move of any contract or partial contract to the value of £50 000 or more. This information is communicated to the relevant provider as the loss of income means they must adjust their own forward planning accordingly. Some FHSAs also ask to be informed of minor shifts of £25 000 or more, because if several practices move monies of that order the effect would be the same as a major shift.

Each year the items included in the fundholding budget are broadened. Practices must read information from RHAs and FHSAs carefully to stay up to date and to evaluate the effect of any additional item on their budget. When new items are included there are often restrictions on the placement of contracts. For example, when community nursing was introduced in April 1993 fundholding practices were obliged to 'block back' to the traditional provider. From April 1994 the contracts may be placed with a different community trust, but nowhere else. Each year the controls are likely to be relaxed, but the fund manager must stay aware of the changing guidelines.

Negotiating Process

When a practice has agreed their budget they can begin the contract negotiation process with providers, although these two priorities are often running simultaneously during January, February and March. An effective contract is one of the basics in fundholding, as without it the service provisions will never move forward in a desirable way for the practice. The contract is a document that includes legal obligations, Patient's Charter rights, financial and quality agreements. The practice can put forward its own contract to the provider for discussion or the provider can put forward their own. It will usually depend upon the practice's satisfaction with the service it receives from each provider, and like so much in fundholding will depend upon discussion and local agreements.

The negotiation process beings long before any meeting with representatives from providers and carries on throughout the financial year, and even into the following year when modifications are needed.

Steps in the negotiating process

1 Preparation.
2 Openings and testing.
3 Concessions and bargaining.
4 Conclusions and agreements.
5 Monitoring and audit.

Preparation
Contracts cannot be effectively negotiated in total, and should be broken down into component parts. Some areas will be acceptable and no changes necessary, but others will be causing concern and these should be analysed to identify exactly what needs to be modified or moved to another provider. This will avoid time being wasted on unimportant details and increase the

chances of leaving the meeting with some progress having been made. Part of the preparation and data collection will arise from the current contract reviews – these could be either clinical or administrative issues. When making a criticism it is always a good idea to have specific examples at hand to illustrate the point. Proper preparation will lead to a set of objectives, although it is unrealistic to expect that they will all be met as the other party may have a conflicting list! For this reason the practice must devise a 'fall-back' position and identify one or two priority objectives and be prepared to compromise on the rest.

Good preparation includes some research into the other party's situation. This information will help to anticipate objections and have comprehensive answers or responses at hand.

Opening and testing

This is the first phase of face to face negotiation with a provider. Time should be spent creating a reasonably harmonious atmosphere and a few minutes spent on introductions and 'small talk' will not be wasted.

To reinforce this positive approach, the interview should begin with an outline of the agenda and identification of the areas of common ground and shared interests. This phase progresses into the testing, that is, verifying the current situation and correcting any inaccurate assumptions. Listening is as important as speaking, because there may be inconsistencies in the other party's statements and full use must be made of these. This is the opportunity to point out the bargaining position of both sides, state your objectives and try to link them with benefits to the other party. This is also the time to clearly state the areas of conflict that require a solution.

Concessions and bargaining

This is definitely the most skilful area of negotiation, and potentially the most rewarding. It brings bargaining into the equation, especially if the preparation phase has highlighted some weaknesses of the provider, or items that they would find desirable. The art is to sound as reasonable as possible, maximize every concession that you are prepared to make and minimize the others. Confirm every concession offered with appreciation and thanks. The point of this phase is to move the other party closer to your list of objectives and away from theirs. To do this use time pressures, humour, assumed disappointment in their unwillingness to compromise, threats and any information that can be used to your own advantage. Either party leaving the discussion would signify total failure, it is much better to identify the stumbling blocks and arrange another meeting at a future date. Grand gestures like storming out of the room are pointless and more akin to a child having a tantrum, especially when a further meeting is inevitable and you have to face the same people again.

Conclusions and agreement

The agreements need to be summarized and confirmed in writing at the end of the negotiations. If the other party has made concessions that were initially stated to be impossible, help them to save face by remaining polite and appreciative. The meeting should end as it began, on a positive note with all parties feeling that they have had adequate opportunities to describe their situation and objectives. If there are one or two unresolved areas these can be delayed for a future interview when further investigations have taken place. This should not prevent the remainder of the agreements going forward to a formal contract arrangement.

Monitoring and audit

At the end of the negotiating process look critically at your own performance and see where it could have been improved. It may be that the other party was a particularly skilful negotiator and things could be learned from their techniques.

Getting issues written into a contract is only half the battle! They must be monitored carefully and dates set for regular review meetings. This will give sufficient time to take corrective action if things are deviating from the original contract.

Monitoring the budget

As stated previously, a fundholder's performance is based on the net over- or under-spend on all elements of the budget. However, to try to monitor a total budget would be difficult and confusing, it is much easier to manage four individual budgets.

At the beginning of the financial year the fundholder will be asked to submit a plan of their target spending and savings and how they intend to achieve them. This helps the practice to prove that they have clear priorities and plans to utilize the budget effectively. Conversely, should the practice feel that their budget is inadequate they can accept it with caveats which may help them to obtain additional funding later in the year if their predictions are correct.

If the fund manager treats each portion of the budget as a separate entity it is simpler to control, and has an obvious impact on the net out-turn. A planned underspend in one area can offset a planned overspend in another. The key is 'planned' and the FHSA will want to see clear evidence that the practice objectives have been borne out by the actions to achieve the intended position at the end of the year. All of the monitoring guidelines, given under *The Preparatory Year* at the start of this chapter, apply equally to monitoring a real budget.

The hospital services element is the most difficult to control because patients' needs do not always conform to the case mix allocated in the budget. Those practices with smaller list sizes are more vulnerable than those with large lists, because the impact of variations is greater. It may take only one expensive procedure to move a practice into an overspend situation, even if their controls have been sound and effective.

At the end of each month the fund manager must close the month on the computer software within a timescale stipulated by the FHSA. This involves closing the referral ledger for a given month and entering figures for staff and drug expenditure. Each system is slightly different and full training should be given on this aspect of the fund manager's role. FHSAs have accounting staff designated to fundholding and they can advise on the statements they wish to receive, as well as answering any queries. To give an accurate assessment of the fund status all the systems work on *accruals*, ie entering activity that the practice knows itself liable to pay onto the system. Hence the importance of entering data from out-going and in-coming mail, and not waiting for an invoice or minimum data set from a provider. The statements are a picture of the money due to be spent in that month, which does not necessarily correspond with the invoices authorized for payment. The practice never receives the total budget, only a twelfth of the staffing budget in cash each month. The rest is held by the FHSA to whom invoices are sent for payment, once they have been fully checked and verified.

Each fundholding computer system produces a variety of reports which must be printed and forwarded to the FHSA for their submission to the RHA. This is a condition of being a fundholding practice, and timely submission of such statements is one of the yardsticks used by the FHSA to judge the practice's efficiency and performance.

What happens if we overspend?

As soon as a practice finds it has overspent it must be a priority to find out why. The monthly statements should be carefully scrutinized and further detailed fund reports and schedules produced to pinpoint exactly how the overspend occurred.

The overspend may be planned, for example, a consultant has doubled the number of operations performed in one month to compensate for being away the next month. The practice may have asked for one particular waiting list to be cleared during a quiet time for the provider, knowing that an under-spend in another element will compensate. When a full explanation has been obtained, the FHSA should be informed, preferably in writing. If the over-spend is likely to continue or worsen the practice will be asked what action it intends to take. This could range from forcing the provider to stick to the original activity as agreed in the contract, to delaying in-patient admission dates until the new financial year. If the overspend is in line with the caveats placed in the budget acceptance document, the FHSA may be in a position to review the level of funding. The priority is to keep the FHSA fully informed at all times as they can offer guidance and moral support when the going gets tough. The onus is on the practice to defend its actions and to demonstrate that all reasonable measures to control the budget have been taken.

What happens if we underspend?

Large underspends will raise as many questions as large overspends, and like overspends the practice must be perfectly clear about the reasons. If the savings were planned then there should be no problem and the practice will be able to utilize such savings to improve patient services. They can be added to the following year budget or used for an approved practice scheme. The practice must produce a detailed plan to spend any savings and submit it to the FHSA for approval, and it must be spent within four years.

Every practice must wait until their annual fundholding accounts have been audited before spending any savings, and these are held by the FHSA until required.

Confidentiality

The safety of confidential patient information is a common concern, especially as administrative and financial staff could have access to clinical letters. The official answer is that all health service employees are bound by the same code of confidentiality and will respect information about individuals. Many providers will send authorization requests for extra contractual referrals without a patient name, and address them to the patient's named GP. All such initiatives should be welcomed, if only to prove that the providers are aware of the need to protect confidential information. Where possible fax machines should not be used for sending clinical letters or any document where a patient could be identified. Like telephones, fax machines can suffer from crossed wires and the information may not end up at the right place. If practices are concerned about auditors having access to patient records to check that a payment made for a procedure has been properly verified, they can offer to have a member of staff on hand to look through the notes for the appropriate letter or discharge summary.

The consortium approach

Negotiate jointly, contract separately

It is common for fundholding practices using the same providers to join forces to increase their negotiating power. It is possible to negotiate jointly but contract separately. The advantage comes in putting additional pressure on a provider to introduce a service that everyone agrees is needed, or to improve a particular aspect of their unit. For example, to reduce the waiting time for an orthopaedic out-patient appointment to nine weeks. The forum would normally include the practice fund managers and fundholding partners to discuss areas of mutual concern, and to agree a course of action. If the forum cannot agree then the consortium will not be effective, and should deal with the situation on an individual practice basis. This type of consortium is advantageous because it can be used to best effect when everyone agrees on a topic, but each practice retains its autonomy if it does not share the majority view. By contracting individually each practice can respond to their patients' needs and ensure that the contract is a fair reflection of these.

Negotiate jointly, contract jointly

Another type of consortium will negotiate and contract jointly, and probably works best where there is only one major provider used by all practices. This consortium will probably have one fund manager for all fundholding practices, with a specific brief to act on their behalf. There must be a high level of agreement and shared views for this to be effective, and a comprehensive written agreement about the ways the contracts are apportioned to each practice. This is essential if the contract performance is to be monitored by each practice, and for them to feel that they have ownership of the decisions taken on their behalf. The fund manager must also be a person who has the respect and confidence of all parties, as well as being totally fair to all practices.

Conclusion

By joining a consortium the fundholding practice will achieve two things, a broader knowledge of other's priorities and problems and increased negotiating power. There must be mutual trust and respect and shared views on major issues for it to be effective.

'Total' fundholding

In October 1993, as part of an initiative by a Regional Health Authority to research new ways of purchasing health care, four general practices in the same town were invited to take a total purchasing budget. The four fundholding practices comprised three first-wave and one third-wave practice, caring in all for 39 000 patients out of a health district population of 276 000.

The town has its own community hospital with a GP ward, three other wards for the elderly mental and infirm, geriatric respite care, and long stay care. There are also out-patient, radiology, physiotherapy, occupational therapy departments and an 18 place day hospital for the elderly. The main provider unit for the town, which takes approximately 85% of its in-patients, lies eight miles away, and some patients are treated in neighbouring districts.

The practices have had a very productive, professional relationship for many decades which has been an essential part of good planning and negotiation. This allows division of labour between the practices when taking on new responsibilities for purchasing. Particular areas for examination include respite and long stay care for the elderly, all emergency admissions, all non-fundholding surgery, extra contractual referrals, accident and emergency attendances, and the establishment of a primary care unit involving both general practice work and the care of the injured at the local community hospital.

Conventional fundholding involves the purchasing of out-patient services, a selection of in-patient surgery, community nursing budgets, drugs prescribing and in-house staff salaries and the employer's National Insurance contributions. Purchasing beyond fundholding means purchasing a host of specialist services which include everything from school nursing to neonatal intensive care, from long term care of patients with learning difficulties to heart transplant patients. A budget based on capitation was agreed with the local District Health Authority with an adjustment for the age structure of the practice and deprivation based on a mathematical scoring system called the Townsend Score. This amounted to £13 192 000 of which £3 500 000 was already dedicated to fundholding. A capitation based budget was requested by the practices in order to lay to rest, at the beginning of the project, any criticism about practices receiving more than their fair share of revenue to purchase services.

Experience of the fundholding practices has been that having contracts with providers which allow payment for each item of work (cost per case) is the most sensitive way for analysing work done against money spent. Furthermore, the accurate recording of activity in each area is vital to track both expenditure and to change future contracts, whilst at the same time receiving an adequate quality of care.

After taking advice a central computer was established in one of the surgeries with a telephone link line to the other three surgeries. A separate staff of four clerks and a manager were appointed to oversee the scheme, and all were responsible through the project manager to the Health Authority, who had overriding rights to abort the scheme at any time and take over the expenditure. The main administrative load would fall on each practice to have written confirmation of all hospital and other activities carried out so that correct input can be made in each of the surgeries relating to work done within the scheme. All savings from the scheme were not to be treated like fundholding savings, which revert exclusively to the practice, but were to be spent on the patients of the town collectively.

Some of the areas to be reviewed include the changing of respite care and long stay care of the elderly from the local community hospital which is a high cost, to ten nursing home beds at a much lower level of cost. Emergency admissions would be closely analysed and their role in admitting elderly patients under the care of their GP rather than a consultant, into nursing homes rather than into hospitals, was investigated. Enhancements of staffing levels within the community will allow the development of a so called 'hospital at home', where early discharge of surgical cases can be undertaken.

The establishment of the local community hospital as a physical base for all community services was planned. A proper primary care unit with a mix of general practice patients and minor injury patients was to be set up. Overall, the philosophy will be that as many services as possible will be provided in the town itself, with the provision of other services to be as near as possible to the locality.

Clearly, this is a highly experimental purchasing scheme which, after two years, should highlight the strengths and shortcomings of a system which allows GPs to influence directly all the purchasing of all the health care services.

11 Managing Patients

To some, the very title of this chapter may seem a misnomer. General practice is, after all, essentially a service led by the demands of patients. Many GPs feel that so much time is spent responding to these demands for care and support that they are unable to cope with any of the other aspects of primary care. Perhaps, for them, 'Managing workload' would be a more appropriate title!

Whilst the treatment of acute illness is undoubtedly an important part of general practice, the development of the primary health care team has made it possible to plan care in a way that benefits both patients and health care workers.

One of the basic principles of the National Health Service has always been that patients should be able to obtain medical advice, when required, free at the point of access. What is often forgotten is that, in order to make proper use of the service and to be able to make sensible decisions about when and how to seek medical advice, patients must have relevant information. In this way they can maintain their independence and retain responsibility for their own health.

The practice manager has a key role in co-ordinating all the activities of primary care, including the dissemination of information. This chapter discusses:

- the legal and contractual obligations of primary care
- the assessment of the needs of patients
- the promotion of the practice as a friendly and helpful organization
- the principles governing the provision of
  - clinical care
  - health education and the prevention of disease.

Rights and duties – the basic service

The general practitioners' contract with the NHS

Whilst the financial arrangements for the general practitioners' contract with the health service are to be found in what is generally referred to as 'The Red

Book', the rules under which GPs work are laid down in the document 'The Terms and Conditions of Service for General Practitioners', published by the National Health Service Executive. Although it is seldom needed, it is important to have an up-to-date copy in the practice.

As patients become more aware of their rights, they tend to complain about their doctors more frequently. A GP these days can expect to have an average of four formal complaints made against him during his medical lifetime. Whilst many minor grievances are dealt with informally by the practice manager, official complaints are made to the Family Health Services Authority (FHSA), whose job it is to see 'fair play' and to administer the general practitioners' contract on behalf of the government.

The majority of complaints are due to misunderstanding and poor communication, and many of these can be settled by the informal procedure arranged by the FHSA. However, when a serious breach of the terms of service appears to have taken place, a formal hearing is likely. In this case, when the GP concerned is informed that a complaint has been made, he or she is sent copies of the correspondence and told which part of the contract may have been broken. The commonest is paragraph 13, part of which reads:

> '. . . a doctor shall render to his patients all necessary and appropriate personal medical services of the type usually provided by general medical practitioners.'

This means that practitioners are not required to know everything or be able to do everything. They are, however, expected to behave as other general practitioners, as a group, would normally be expected to behave! In other words, offending doctors will be judged against the performance of their peers.

There is no need to go into detail about the complaints procedure here, but it is important to point out that awaiting the hearing of a complaint is an extremely stressful experience for all concerned – patients and doctors alike. A practice manager who is aware of this can help the doctor concerned by:

- acting as a good listener
- checking the necessary paperwork
- making sure that the partner under threat is adequately supported
  - by family, friends and partners
  - by a representative from the local medical committee, Royal College of General Practitioners or other organization
  - by his or her defence society, if necessary.

The Patients' Charter

In March 1993 the Department of Health and the Central Office of Information published 'The Patient's Charter – and the family doctor services'.
Although it was written for the purpose of raising the standards of general
practice, it does, of course, describe only a set of minimal requirements. It
states that every person in the country has the right:

- to be registered with a family doctor
- to change doctor quickly and easily
- to be *offered* a health check when joining a doctor's list for the first time,
  or at home, yearly, if 75 years old or over
- to receive *emergency care* at any time through a family doctor
- to have *appropriate* drugs and medicine prescribed
- to be referred to an acceptable consultant when the family doctor thinks
  necessary, and to be referred for a second opinion *if the patient and family
  doctor think it desirable*
- to have access to personal medical records, *subject to any limitations by
  law*
- to know that those working for the NHS are under a legal duty to keep
  the contents of health records confidential
- to choose whether or not to take part in medical research or student
  training
- to be given detailed information about local family doctor services
  through the local FHSA's directory
- to receive a copy of the doctor's practice leaflet, setting out the services
  he or she provides
- to receive a full and prompt reply to any complaint made about NHS
  services.

(*Source*: Leaflet HP13. Department of Health, March 1993)

Although at first sight the Charter appears one sided (it makes no mention
of the patient's responsibilities), it is, in fact, quite reasonable, especially when
you consider the sections in italics. Some of the points raised will be
considered in more detail later.

The Charter also recommends that FHSAs should encourage practices to
set their own standards for such things as availability, waiting times and the
issue of repeat prescriptions but, as GPs are private contractors to the health
service, their involvement in this initiative is purely voluntary. However,
many surgeries have chosen to create their own criteria and publish them in
their information leaflets and practice reports.

The practice leaflet

This is an important way of informing patients about the way the practice works, and it is worth while spending time and money in order to produce clear and attractively designed leaflets. They may stand behind many a clock on many a mantelpiece for many a year, but they will be seen by a great many people and form a valuable part of their first impressions of the practice. Under the terms of service, certain information must be included. The list below more than covers this requirement.

- Names, qualifications and year of birth or first qualification of doctor(s).
- Surgery times.
- Information about making appointments.
- Arrangements for home visits.
- Emergency call procedures.
- Off-duty arrangements.
- Repeat prescription (and dispensing) arrangements.
- Clinic times.
- Details of staff employed.
- Other services.
- Patient participation activities.
- The geographical area covered by the practice.
- Access for the disabled.

Source: Health Department 1990 Contract

Access to health records

Over the last few years a number of legal changes have taken place that allow patients increased access to their medical records and, although this has not altered the way patients behave, it has certainly changed the way in which medical practitioners write their notes! Gone are the days when a doctor could write pithy comments about his own feelings or his patient's behaviour. 'Haematomentia', 'ossilatum plumbum' and ' 'Urts' ere's syndrome' are now conditions of the past!

It is important for a practice manager to have a working knowledge of recent legislation in order to advise patients, receptionists and doctors, and be able to institute appropriate procedures in the practice.

Summary of legislation

Data Protection Act 1984
Although certain information is exempt, section 21 of this Act allows patients access to their computerized health records.

Access to Personal Files Act 1987

This gives individuals a right of access to records not held on computer (so-called 'manual records'), including those held by local authorities, social services and other agencies.

Access to Medical Reports Act 1988

This provides that an employer or insurance company cannot seek a medical report on an individual from the doctor responsible for that individual's care and treatment, without that individual's knowledge and consent. The person concerned also has the right to see the report before it is passed to the employer/insurance company, may then request that corrections be made, and ultimately has the right to refuse to allow the report to be passed on to the employer/insurance company.

Access to Health Records Act 1990

The effect of this Act is really the same as the Data Protection Act and extends the established principles and procedures of patient access to cover all health records *compiled on or after November 1991*. This Act sets out the procedures that individuals must follow to apply for access, the relevant time limits within which a response has to be made, and the changes that can be made to those records if the patient believes them to be inaccurate.

Needs and wants

The contractual arrangements of medical practice are the lowest denominators of care and, as such, form only the basis on which a good manager will seek to build a quality service. In order to do this, it is necessary to balance availability against demand, to recognize the needs of individuals as well as those of the practice community, and to weigh them against the resources and capabilities of the practice team. Instead of responding to patient demand, a good manager must try to identify 'needs', as opposed to 'wants', and provide an appropriate service. How can this difficult task be done?

Consumerism – 'needs' assessment

Practice statistics

'Needs' assessment can take place all the time, as patients use the system and the team responds to changes in workload. The introduction of the computer has made it easy to collect basic data on such items as the weekly totals of consultations and visits, the numbers attending clinics, and so on. The usefulness of this type of information increases as patterns of attendance emerge. For example, it becomes possible for a manager to predict workload and approach the doctors to say, 'With Dr X away, we need to find 70 extra appointments next week – thus enabling decisions to be made concerning the provision of these appointments.

Informal 'feedback'

On the whole, when asked, patients tend to say nice things about their practice. After all, nobody wishes to make themselves unpopular! Often, however, they will drop valuable hints about the service provided and everyone should be prepared to listen to what they have to say. Attached staff are more likely to hear the truth than doctors, and patients' comments can be useful in deciding which aspects of the practice to investigate further.

Surveys of patient opinion

Questionnaires
These can be very useful for finding the answers to specific questions. The questionnaire should be short, easy to answer and, perhaps more importantly, easy to analyse. Time spent in design and preparation, with the advice of someone with experience, is time well spent. It is also sensible to try the questionnaire out on a few patients before issuing it in large numbers. Surprisingly often, it is found that a silly or confusing question has been included on the form without the designer realizing it!

Structured interviews
Ideally, these should be carried out by someone from outside the practice. Using an agreed structure, the interviewer promotes discussion on a series of predetermined topics, recording opinions as the interview progresses. Conducted with randomly selected individuals drawn from various age or interest groups, this method tends to be expensive to administer. However, although the samples are usually small, the method can provide very useful insights into how the work of the practice is perceived.

For example, a recent survey of this type in my own practice highlighted the following.

- The importance placed by patients on getting an appointment quickly. [As might be expected.]
- The fact that the practice record was good in this respect, but that the hours of availability were not right for some working people. [Reassuring, but more information is needed before any changes can be considered.]
- The need for improved telephone access to the doctors for advice. [A good idea which is being investigated.]
- Appreciation of the new health promotion clinics. [Perhaps not a wasted effort after all!]

- The need for the doctors to make known their views on complementary medicine. [A surprise.]

Suggestions boxes

Whilst these are a recognized feature of most surgeries, many find that they seldom produce anything other than occasional humorous comments or violent abuse.

Patient participation

This is a useful way of harnessing the tremendous goodwill that undoubtedly exists among patients. When working well, such a group can represent the views of the practice community. Finding the right 'mix' of people in order to represent all sections of the practice population can be difficult. At its best, it can have a constructive influence on the development of the practice; at its worst, it can be dominated by well-meaning busybodies or become a tool for 'rubber stamping' the doctors' views.

Such a group should be able to give the practice advice on, for example:

- facilities such as play areas and pram parks
- surgery hours and appointment systems
- clinics and out-of-hours services
- additional services such as chiropody, physiotherapy, etc.

Finally, the group may form a focus for fund raising for the purchase of equipment, or take on responsibility for the development of some services themselves, such as visiting the elderly and transporting them to and from the shops or surgery.

Having gathered all the information about the patient's needs and compared it with what is already being done, the practice manager should then make plans to modify or develop the services on offer. Any planned developments must be consistent with the overall philosophy and objectives of the practice. Before making any changes, it is important that everyone in the practice understands and agrees with what is being suggested. Perhaps the best way to do this is to develop a set of aims and objectives for the practice, as discussed in Chapters 3 and 4.

The practice image

Having listened to the patients' views and, as far as possible, taken them into account, what better way can there be of creating a good impression than by informing them of your plans – by advertising your services and by making your standards of care explicit?

Advertising

In the past, doctors were not permitted to advertise; indeed, the General Medical Council (GMC), which governs the professional behaviour of doctors, still lays down strict guidelines. However, in line with the government's wish to improve the service by increasing competition, some of the restrictions have been relaxed recently, and it is now permissible to make factual information available to the public.

At present, most practices restrict their activities in this area to the production of a practice leaflet (described earlier) containing information about the services provided. It is important to make sure that the information contained in any advertisement is accurate, and that, whilst it describes the range of services available, it does not disparage other practices by suggesting superior skills.

Accessibility and availability

The reputation of the practice as a friendly and helpful organization is far more important than any glossy brochure, and time spent considering this will not be wasted. Carry out a hypothetical test on your own practice by answering the following questions.

Mrs Whittle is worried, but she thinks that if she could talk to the doctor for a minute or two, she might be reassured.

1 Can she find the practice telephone number? (Is it clearly given in the telephone directory, the Yellow Pages and the practice leaflet?)
2 Does she know that there is a special time to telephone when she will be able to get advice from her own GP?
3 When she telephones, is the line always engaged? (Does the surgery have enough lines?)
4 How does the receptionist answer the telephone? (Does she sound friendly? Has she had any training on how to answer and deal with anxious people?)

Mrs Whittle's doctor is helpful, but thinks she should be seen.

5 Does the surgery have a policy for urgent appointments? Are there any appointments set aside each day for late bookings? Will her 'own' doctor be able to see her, or will she perhaps be given an appointment with another partner or with the trainee?

Mrs Whittle arrives at the surgery.

6 How does the receptionist greet her? Does she smile, even at the end of a long day?

Mrs Whittle's doctor is running late.

7 Are the patients in the waiting room informed of the reason for any prolonged delays? Does the doctor greet Mrs Whittle personally and apologize when she enters the consulting room?

If he does, Mrs Whittle may well feel rather special at being 'fitted in' when her doctor is so busy, and she will undoubtedly tell her friends what a considerate practice she belongs to!

Questions 1 and 3 above concern *accessibility*, i.e. the ease with which the patients can avail themselves of the service.

Question 5 is about a particular doctor's *availability*, i.e. whether the doctor is around when needed, or always off writing books or at meetings!

Question 2 concerns *information and advertising*, whilst questions 4, 6, and 7 all contribute to the *practice image* and are probably just as important as a warm comfortable waiting room with up-to-date magazines, although these should not be forgotten.

Some of the factors that influence accessibility are obviously outside the practice's control; for example, bus services, car ownership and the availability of public telephones. Others, such as parking spaces, ramps for the disabled and surgery design, can be considered only when planning improvements to the building or moving to new premises. However, telephones, appointment systems, surgery hours and other activities affected by workload can be modified to suit local demand. It is here that the practice manager must negotiate a compromise between the demands of patients and the interests of the doctors, receptionist and attached staff.

Surveys that have been conducted on the satisfaction of patients with primary care services consistently show that what the public appreciate is:

- quick access to medical advice
- a simple, friendly and efficient service
- a doctor who listens, is interested and explains.

To this must now be added good basic health education for the prevention of disease. It is interesting that patients take basic safety and efficient emergency care for granted, but do not necessarily expect their GP to be brilliant or clever (although most agree that it helps!).

Systems and procedures

No efficient service can exist without good organization, and all organizations require administration. Office systems and procedures must be carefully designed with the advice of those involved. Procedures, once agreed, should be recorded, preferably in a way that allows for audit and subsequent modification. Many practices collect their written procedures in a book which can then be referred to at any time. This promotes confidence and consistent behaviour among the staff.

Recall, registers and review

A look at Mrs Whittle's medical records reveals why she is such a worrier. There is a strong history of heart disease in her family. Her doctor has recorded this in her notes, but does the practice have a system that would identify her special risk and ensure that appropriate action is taken?

These matters are, of course, more properly the province of the doctors, and computerization has made the identification and follow-up of patients much easier. However, a practice manager should be involved in the administration of the procedures. The practice manager should:

- help the partners and the nursing team to design protocols for preventive care and disease management that fit into the other work of the practice
- decide, with the practice staff, on the procedures for administering the protocols and clinics
- monitor the results by arranging the collection of statistics on such items as attendance figures and long-term medication.

A recent survey in our practice showed that patients appreciated the increased emphasis on health education and prevention, brought about by the introduction of the new contract for general practitioners. One might argue about the effectiveness of such programmes on scientific grounds, but there can be no doubt that the exercise of providing such a service encourages teamwork, generates confidence and trust in both patients and staff, and demonstrates that the practice is interested in the welfare of its patients.

Confidentiality

Confidentiality is the cornerstone of trust. Patients trust doctors and, to a large extent, extend that trust to the whole of the primary health care team. In general, attached staff – nurses, health visitors, community psychiatric nurses and qualified counsellors – are bound by the same rules of confidentiality as doctors and, as such, are often given access to the patient's complete medical records. Receptionists and other staff who need access to this information in order to perform their duties must also be bound by the same rules.

Doctors have a habit of discussing problem cases over coffee, and often let off steam after a long and trying day. Receptionists and other staff may overhear some of these outbursts which, on occasion, may even involve someone they know. They *must* understand the rule that 'what goes on here, stays here!' This principle is so important that, in most practices, a breach of confidence by a member of staff is one of the few things that will result in instant dismissal. It is wise to make this quite clear at the beginning of a person's employment and issue periodic reminders thereafter.

Staff also need to be trained not to let information slip unintentionally. Most realize that it would be wrong to tell Auntie Flo' the result of her niece's pregnancy test, but few understand that to confirm to a husband that his wife has an appointment might be a technical breach of confidence. Although a slip of this sort seldom matters, it is best to have strict rules regarding the release of information to anyone other than the patient concerned. All staff should be encouraged to develop total amnesia about what has gone on in the practice as soon as they leave work!

The need to know

Most computer systems, by using 'passwords', have the facility of restricting access to varying levels of information. The security of medical records should therefore improve as the right of access is confined to those who 'need to know'. For example, there will be some instances where it will be in the patient's best interests for a counsellor or social worker to have access to selected medical information, but this is by no means always the case. Practice managers need to be aware of this fact and to make sure that it is reflected in the practice procedures for access to records.

Equipment and supplies

Having the right tools for a job can make all the difference to the quality of a final product. The purchase of equipment and the maintenance of supplies is an important management function which is dealt with elsewhere (*see* Chapter 9). Good managers will have check lists and procedures to ensure that the consulting and treatment areas do not run out of essential supplies. They will also be in a position to help with the purchase of equipment – for example, for a new treatment room. The manager will need to know the size of the budget set aside for the purpose, obtain catalogues and, having helped the partners and practice nurses decide on their priorities, will then be in a position to order the chosen equipment and oversee the project in general.

Conclusion

This chapter has considered the administration and management of patient care:

- contractual obligations – the minimum standards
- needs assessment – how to gather the information needed for planning services
- the organization of services – the achievement of optimum standards by balancing what is required against what is available
- the creation of an environment that is regarded as accessible, friendly and efficient – publicity and public relations

The chapter began by suggesting that the title 'Managing Patients' was perhaps inappropriate and that 'Managing Workload' might be more accurate. However, this title is also rather one sided as it suggests that the object of the exercise is solely to control the patients' behaviour for the benefit of the practice. Later in the chapter, the balance between 'needs', 'wants' and 'possibilities' was explored. This balancing of the needs of the patients on the one hand and the practice team on the other is one of the most difficult but fascinating tasks of the practice manager.

Planning is an integral part of practice management, but the unexpected can , and frequently does, happen. Although to some extent it can be allowed for, it can never be planned! It is the 'unexpected' that puts any system, however efficient, under strain and it is then that the flexibility and goodwill of doctors, patients and staff are required. You cannot please all the people all the time, so perhaps the title of this chapter should be 'Managing *for* People'.

References

The terms of service for doctors in general practice. Department of Health, London.

The patient's charter. Department of Health, London.

The 1990 contract. Department of Health, London.

Access to Health Records Act 1990. NHS Management Executive.

Pritchard P. Patient participation in primary health care. In: *Doctor–patient communication*, eds D. Pendleton and J. Hasler. Academic Press, London, 1992.

Professional conduct and discipline: fitness to practice. General Medical Council, London, 1992.

– Guide to NHS complaints. *Which?* April 1993.
– Getting to see your GP. *Which?* March 1993.

For Reference and Further Reading

Hasler J, Bryceland C, Hobden-Clarke L and Rose P. *Handbook of practice management.* Churchill Livingstone, Edinburgh, 1993

Hasler J and Schofield T, eds. *Continuing care: the management of chronic disease*, 2nd edn. Oxford University Press, Oxford, 1990

Buckley G. Auditing the organisation. In: *Medical audit and general practice*, ed M Marinker. Published for the MSD Foundation by the British Medical Journal, London, 1990

Pritchard P. The management of prevention. In: *Prevention in general practice*, 2nd edn, eds G Fowler, JAM Gray and P Anderson. Oxford University Press, Oxford, 1993

12 Managing Prescribing

THE act of prescribing a medicine for a patient is an exceptionally complex procedure. Not only is it the second most important therapeutic tool the doctor possesses – the first is the listening ear – but also the reasons for seeking and issuing a prescription are many and varied. Most commonly a prescription is issued because the patient has a disease or a problem that the doctor considers likely to respond to that treatment. At other times, the process of issuing the prescription is itself the therapeutic part of the transaction and up to 40% of symptoms will be alleviated by a placebo. Yet again, a patient may seek a prescription as a way of maintaining contract with the surgery and sometimes does not take the tablets or even get the prescription filled. Sometimes a doctor will use a prescription as a way of ensuring that a patient returns for review, and at other times may deem it more helpful to accede to an illogical request from a patient rather than damage an important relationship.

Yet economy and efficiency are of crucial importance to the National Health Service, for general practice accounts for 11% of the total budget; in 1991/92 the rate of increase in expenditure was over 12% – much greater than the rate of inflation. Some of this increase was because of the advent of new, effective and more expensive drugs but much cannot be explained by this and probably represents both an increased patient demand for care and a lack of good control by doctors. This latter explanation is given credence by the extreme variation in drug expenditure by individual GPs, which can amount to as much as a threefold difference between doctors. There is also much evidence of over-prescribing and inappropriate prescribing* revealed by the number of patients, particularly the elderly, admitted to hospital with iatrogenic disease and the reduction in cost achieved when doctors analyse their prescribing carefully. The Department of Health, and many doctors, feel that this is an area where considerable savings can be made, and set a target increase in expenditure for 1993/94 of only 6.35%. This has effectively put a stop to what previously was a non cash limited budget for GP prescribing.

*See also The Audit Commission's report 'A Prescription for Improvement' HMSO

Prescribing and the law

A practice manager will want to ensure that all the staff are familiar with the requirements of the law and those of the NHS relating to the prescribing of medicine. There is no better source of information about this than that set out in the first 14 pages or so of the British National Formulary. This repays careful study and also outlines the important responsibilities relating to the reporting of adverse reactions to drugs and the special regulations about Controlled Drugs and their safe-keeping. It goes without saying that the same security requirements for drugs applies to the prescriptions for those drugs.

Practice formularies

There are something like 7500 individual preparations available on prescription. Many of these are the same drug in a different formulation or just with a different proprietary name but they still provide the doctor and practice with a formidable range from which to choose. In fact, individual doctors limit their choice to just under 200 preparations, but within a group practice this may still mean that 300–400 preparations form the list of chosen drugs. Whilst it would be desirable to limit this to a smaller number in order that everyone became familiar with the characteristics of each drug, it is not easy. Patients bring their own 'list' from other practices, individuals have idiosyncratic responses to drugs and doctors from different generations have been brought up to use different drugs. Nevertheless, it is desirable to reduce the range as much as possible, and practices will use guidelines and practice formularies in an attempt to achieve a rational approach.

Sometimes these formularies will be 'borrowed' from another source (the Lothian and the Northern Ireland Faculties of the Royal College of General Practitioners have produced particularly useful examples) but often a practice or a group of local practices will set out to create their own formulary. There is much to commend this exercise for the educational effect of having to make a choice and consider pharmacological action, potential adverse effects, differing formulations and cost is considerable. However, the time taken to do this work is great and many practices start out on the exercise and subsequently abandon it before completion. Nevertheless, even the rationalization of choice within a single therapeutic group can be a very stimulating intellectual exercise.

Sources of information include *British National Formulary*, MIMS (Monthly Index of Medical Specialities), *Martindale's Pharmacopoeia* (published by the Pharmaceutical Society of Great Britain), *Treatment* (published by Churchill Livingstone) and now a number of computerized drug databases that may form part of a practice's database in the future.

Controlling prescribing

There was previously an open-ended commitment from the NHS to pay for all the drugs prescribed, with the exception of the contribution towards the cost paid by a minority of patients, without any restriction upon the individual doctor except for a visit, to give advice, from the Regional Medical Service in the case of persistent over-prescribing. In fact, this was surprisingly effective but a more rational solution was sought. The first step was to provide each doctor with up-to-date information about his or her prescribing, together with the cost, so that comparisons could be made and economies sought by individuals and groups of doctors.

Prescribing analysis and cost (PACT)

Each quarter every partner in a practice, or single-handed doctor, is sent details of his or her prescribing for the previous quarter and that of the whole practice by the Prescription Pricing Authority (PPA). The data are derived from all the prescriptions presented to the PPA for payment by retail pharmacists and dispensing doctors. In these reports the total cost is compared with a notional FHSA and national average. It is sent to individuals in order to maintain confidentiality but of course most group practices share the information. Information is also presented on the number of items prescribed, the average cost of items, the percentage of generic prescribing; these data are then broken down into major therapeutic groups so that each of these, say drugs for the cardiovascular system, can be looked at separately.

This information, Level 1, is sent to all doctors without their having to make a request, and it provides useful but fairly basic facts about the quantity of prescribing. In order to consider the quality of prescribing, more data with more detailed analysis of it are required. This information can be obtained by requesting Level 2 data. This provides details to the practice of the prescribing of the six highest cost drugs in each therapeutic group. It thus allows a practice to look at the areas of greatest expense. As well as being supplied on request, it is sent automatically to any practice whose prescribing cost is either 25% above the FHSA average for all prescribing or 75% above the average cost in one of the six major therapeutic groups. It thus allows this difference to be examined to ascertain whether a reduction is possible.

Finally, data are also available at Level 3. These reports contain details of every prescription the doctor or the practice has had dispensed during the previous three months. They are detailed and bulky and are designed to allow rigorous scrutiny for purposes such as the construction of a practice formulary or an audit or the preparation of prescribing protocols within the practice. Most practices have found it possible to be overwhelmed by the quantity of data in Level 3 and confine their activity to looking at one or two therapeutic groups in any particular quarter.

Drug budgets and indicative prescribing amounts

A further way in which control over excessive expenditure on prescribing is exercised is by giving each fundholding practice a drug budget and each non-fundholding practice an indicative prescribing amount (IPA) each year.

Fundholders

The FHSA responsible for the practice will produce a drug budget for initial discussion with the practice, usually in January. Until now (1993/94), IPAs and drug budgets have been set largely on a historical basis. For 1993/94 the calculation was based on the practice's actual spending on drugs for the period 1 April 1992 to 30 September 1992. There is, however, to be a move over the next three to five years to a weighted capitation method based on 'ASTRO PUs', devised by Professor Conrad Harris; Prescribing Research Unit, Leeds University.

'ASTRO PUs' stand for Age, Sex, Temporary Resident Orientated Pre-scribing Units, and these are calculated according to the categories shown in Table 11.1. Clearly this would be too crude a calculation to provide a fair drug budget or IPA, so it will be necessary to add other factors such as significant demographic elements or the fact that a practice is responsible for a large institution for epileptics or young severely disabled people. It will also be necessary still to keep track of the prescribing of expensive medicines.

Final agreement should be reached by the end of March before the new prescribing year begins on 1 April. This figure then becomes the real budget and any savings made by more economical prescribing can be used by the

Table 12.1 Calculation of ASTRO prescribing units

Age	Male PU value	Female PU value
0–4	1	1
5–14	1	1
15–24	1	2
25–34	1	2
35–44	2	3
45–54	3	4
55–64	6	6
65–74	10	10
75+	10	12
Temporary residents	0.5	0.5

practice either to offset over-spending on the staff or hospital budgets or to improve the services and facilities of the practice as approved under the fundholding arrangements.

Non-fundholders

The scheme for non-fundholders has become rather similar to that for fundholders. An IPA is produced by the FHSA that the practice is invited to accept. Initially there was no penalty for exceeding the amount and no reward for making savings but there is now an incentive scheme for non-fundholders that may enhance its cost-effectiveness. This is being arranged on a regional basis to provide non-fundholders with a small financial reward for keeping below their IPA. In the Oxford region, for example, the proposed scheme is that any practice that achieves at least a 1% saving below their IPA will be allowed to keep 20% and 50% of any further savings up to a maximum of £3 000 per partner for use in their own practice.

Both these schemes have to be managed by the practice. The PPA send each practice a monthly statement to enable them to monitor progress throughout the year. The statements are sent about one month in arrears, and the following example shows the sort of information they provide:

Annual amount (agreed budget or IPA)	£488 132
Expenditure for the previous month	£35 972
Cumulative expenditure for the year	£419 939
Projected annual out-turn based on last year's expenditure pattern	£463 509

Obviously the last figure has to be compared with the first to see if there is likely to be an under- or over-spend at the end of the year; in this example the practice is heading for a healthy under-spend.

The role of the practice manager could be to present these figures to the practice together with the associated data from the PPA which give the monthly and cumulative breakdown of expenditure by major therapeutic group and the annual profile of the current and previous monthly figures for comparative purposes. The practice will want the data analysed to see whether any changes in prescribing policy are required, any additional information from PACT about drug usage needed or any additional information about therapeutic alternatives sought.

FHSA professional advisers

All FHSAs have appointed Medical and, in most cases, Pharmaceutical Advisers. There may also be a Pharmaceutical Facilitator whose role is to work with practices encouraging more rational prescribing. Cynics may say that these people are only there to help ration prescribing but in fact they are just as concerned with under-prescribing, for example in the under-use of inhaled steroids in the management of asthma or Angiotensin converting enzyme inhibitors (ACEI) in heart failure. They are helped by the use of an on-line link between the FHSA and the PPA, called Pactline. At present this allows only Level 2 data for a practice to be scrutinized but shortly it will allow scrutiny of data at Level 3 and this will then permit the identification of the times when expensive medicines are started and stopped by a practice, thus relieving them of the burden of having to report all these to the FHSA.

Repeat prescribing

Within the statement of Fees and Allowances there is a requirement that a practice reports on the method it uses for managing repeat prescribing. It is an area of practice management that produces problems, for it requires a very careful and exact level of control whilst providing an element of flexibility to fit in with patient's varied needs. Some repeat prescriptions are handwritten by receptionists and this can, in theory, cause problems because practice staff may not know the implications of what they are writing. Some practices still do not have an automatic check system that prevents patients collecting prescriptions without ever seeing a doctor, and yet others do not have reliable ways in which handwritten prescriptions get into the practice notes. The criteria for an effective system are shown in Table 12.2.

The great majority of prescriptions are now computer produced. For those still written manually the system should fit these criteria, and this should cover those practices that are not fully computerized and those few manually produced prescriptions that are still needed within a fully computerized practice.

There is potential within the increasing role of the community pharmacist to help practices with the monitoring of repeat prescribing and their membership of the Primary Health Care Team should be welcomed.

Table 12.2:   Repeat prescribing system objectives.

1	Prescriptions should be obtainable within 24 hours of ordering
2	Prescriptions should be produced with meticulous accuracy without errors
3	There should be a built-in repeat recall system
4	The clinical records should show what drugs are being taken and when the last supply was obtained
5	The system should be as simple as possible
6	The system should enable audit to be carried out
7	It should be possible to check patient compliance

13 Health and Safety

THE duties of an employer arising from the Health and Safety at Work Act 1974 are not difficult to understand or to apply. Most surgery premises should meet the Act's requirements and its regulations; apart from some minor technical matters there is little in the legislation that should worry a GP or practice manager.

Surgery premises are included in the 'health services' grouping and they are inspected by an official of the Health and Safety Executive (HSE) and not, as often assumed, by a local government environmental officer. HSE inspectors visit GP surgeries from time to time, and the frequency of these visits is increasing. This chapter provides guidance on those matters that an HSE inspector may discuss with the practice manager and her staff. It does not provide a definitive statement or interpretation of the legislation.

The legislation requires an employer, including a self-employed person, to provide and maintain a safe working environment. The Act has established powers and penalties to enforce safety laws. Like most employment legislation, this law pays little regard to the limited resources of a small employer. Many of its provisions are aimed at companies where trade unions are recognized. For instance, the law states that union safety representatives and safety committees should be appointed if these are requested by a recognized union. However, even a GP who employs only a handful of staff with no union members has important duties under this Act.

The employer's duties to his staff

The main aim of the Act is to make both employers and employees conscious of the need for safety in all aspects of the day-to-day working environment. The most important duties are those that any employer must fulfil to his staff:

'It shall be the duty of every employer to ensure, so far as is reasonably practicable, the health, safety and welfare at work of all his employees.'
Health and Safety at Work Act 1974

Thus every employer must do all that is reasonably practicable to ensure the well-being of his employees.

What does 'reasonably practicable' mean?

The meaning of 'reasonably practicable' can be drawn from case law and the advice of HSE inspectors. Any proceedings taken under the Act are criminal, and any employee can report to the HSE a breach of an employer's statutory duty. The HSE may then bring criminal charges.

A court's assessment of whether it was 'reasonably practicable' to avoid a particular hazard or risk of injury takes account of the cost of preventative action (particularly if the employer has few staff and limited resources) and weighs this against the risk of injury and its possible severity. Thus in general practice, a larger practice would carry a heavier burden of responsibility than one with fewer staff and resources.

It is not enough to ensure that equipment and methods of working are safe. Safe systems of working need to be understood and applied by all staff.

Written statement of safety policy

The law requires an employer to provide information, training and supervision for staff on health and safety matters. Unless there are fewer than five staff, the employer must provide a statement of general policy on health and safety and arrangements for implementing this. Employees should be consulted about the form and content of this statement.

The HSE discourage the use of 'model' statements. They believe that each employer should prepare his own, because anyone who takes the easy option of adopting a 'model' statement is unlikely to give sufficient thought to his policy and its consequences. However, contrary to this advice, a specimen format for the written statement is in Box 13.2.

When a GP prepares his own 'written statement' it should be simple and concise. Long sentences and long words reduce impact. Any safety rules should be clear and comprehensive.

The written statement may be included in each employee's written contract of employment. If it is included, it may need to be reviewed and amended from time to time and it must apply to everyone working on the surgery premises. In a small practice, with fewer than five staff, the statement can be posted in a public place. It is not necessary to give everyone a copy of the written statement.

Box 13.1: The Health and Safety at Work Act 1974

The Act requires equipment and methods of working to be safe and without risk to health. Attention should be paid to waste-bins, electric typewriters, sterilizers, photocopying machines, heating equipment, computing, furniture, fire extinguishers, electrical plugs and points, light switches, and any other equipment that may be hazardous. The maintenance and renewal of equipment is particularly important. HSE inspectors look at arrangements for regular servicing, eg maintenance contracts for typewriters, servicing contracts for fire extinguishers, and also the age, reliability and positioning of equipment.

Safety officers

Safety officers and safety representatives are appointed if an employer recognizes a trade union. In general practice these are most likely to be found in health centres where health authority staff work alongside practice staff.

Staff who are appointed as safety representatives have considerable powers on health and safety matters: inspecting the workplace, enquiring into accidents, raising complaints directly with the GP and insisting on a joint staff-management safety committee being formed. Safety representatives have a legal right to challenge the employer on all matters relating to health and safety.

It has been proposed that safety representatives and safety committees should be appointed where the staff are not unionized. Because both the employer and staff share a legal duty to promote the health and safety of everyone using the premises, the Health and Safety Commission have suggested that both should be involved in developing and promoting health and safety policy and procedures.

A safety committee is simply not possible in a small practice. Instead, one member of staff could serve as the 'safety officer' to monitor health and safety. The practice manager may be well suited to do this. However, the GPs, as employers, cannot and must not simply pass over their responsibility as employers to the practice manager. They must be involved and the 'safety officer' should report to one of the partners.

Duties to other persons using the premises

Whilst the Health and Safety Act is mostly concerned with the safety of employees, an employer also has a duty to ensure the safety of anyone who

---

Box 13.2: A specimen written statement on safety

Health and safety in the practice

The partners' policy on health and safety on the surgery premises is to ensure that your working environment is as safe and healthy as possible. As a member of the staff you are expected to support this aim.

Your employer is ultimately responsible for your health and safety; you also have a legal duty to take reasonable care to avoid any action or working pattern that might cause injury to yourself, your colleagues or other people using the surgery premises. In particular, you should not meddle with or misuse any clothing or equipment that has been provided to protect health and safety.

There are certain hazards that you should know about:

1   prams and cycles parked on the premises;
2   medical equipment and instruments used in the consulting rooms;
3   cooking utensils and equipment used in the staff rest room.

You must report any accident to the doctor in charge as soon as possible. You should then write down what has happened, explaining how the accident occurred, so that we can take steps to prevent its repetition.

---

enters the surgery or health centre. This includes patients, pharmaceutical representatives, visitors, builders, tradesmen and health authority staff.

If the premises are owned by a private landlord or local health authority, the licence or lease may impose this duty upon these other parties who may also be liable if there is an accident.

The Act requires the practice to be organized so as to ensure that all users of the premises are safe from risks of personal injury; for example, it is necessary to consider whether they present any potential hazards to elderly or infirm patients. The Occupier's Liability Act 1957 already lays down a 'common duty of care' owed to all persons using the premises.

Notifying accidents and dangerous occurrences

The Act requires the employer to maintain a record of accidents and, if he is the 'controller of the premises', to notify the HSE of certain serious accidents to anyone on the premises, including staff, patients, workmen or health authority staff.

Normally the employer and controller of the premises will be responsible for any accident. Although there may be circumstances where the owner of the premises and not the GPs will be responsible, it is best to assume that the practice should notify the HSE.

COSHH regulations

The Control of Substances Hazardous to Health Regulations 1988 (COSHH) apply obligations on employers to control hazardous substances and to protect people exposed to them. These Regulations cover virtually all substances hazardous to health. Only those substances covered by their own legislation are excluded, such as asbestos, lead and material producing ionizing radiations. The Regulations set out essential measures that employers (and sometimes employees) have to take. Failure to comply with COSHH, in addition to exposing employees to risks, constitutes an offence and is subject to penalties under the Health and Safety at Work Act 1974. Substances hazardous to health include those labelled as dangerous (ie every toxic, harmful, irritant or corrosive) under other statutory requirements.

What are employers required to do?

The basic principles of occupational hygiene underlie the COSHH regulations. These include:

- assessing the risk to health, arising from work and what precautions are needed
- introducing measures to prevent or control the risk
- ensuring that control measures are used, equipment is properly maintained and procedures observed
- monitoring, where necessary, the exposure of employees and carrying out an appropriate form of surveillance of health
- informing, instructing and training employees about the risks and the precautions to be taken.

All employers need to consider how COSHH applies to their employees and working environment. For most GPs compliance should be simple and straightforward. Several publications giving more detailed information on COSHH and its requirements are available from your local office of the HSE.

New health and safety regulations

Six new sets of health and safety at work regulations came into force on 1 January 1993. They apply to virtually all kinds of work activity, including general practice. Like the existing health and safety law, the new regulations place a duty on employers to protect both their employees and other persons, including members of the public.

The new regulations have been introduced to both implement EC Directives and update existing law; they cover:

- general health and safety management
- work equipment safety
- manual handling of loads
- workplace conditions
- personal protective equipment
- display screen equipment.

Most of the duties laid down by the regulations are not completely new; they merely clarify and make more explicit existing health and safety law. Any practice that is already complying with the Health and Safety at Work Act and its regulations should have no difficulty with the new regulations. You may, however, have to take account of some new approaches, especially in relation to managing health and safety and using VDUs.

General health and safety management

These regulations set out general duties that apply to all practices, and are aimed at improving health and safety management. If you are already thorough in your approach to your duties under the Health and Safety at Work (HSW) Act, they should not cause any problems. The regulations require all employers to:

- assess the risk to the health and safety of employees and anyone else affected by your work activity, in order to identify any necessary preventive and protective measures. Employers with five or more employees should write down this risk assessment. (This same threshold already applies in the HSW Act: employers with five or more employees have to prepare a written safety policy)
- arrange for the preventive and protective measures that follow from your risk assessment to be implemented: they should cover planning, organization, control, monitoring and review (ie the management of health and safety). Again, any practice with five or more employees (do not forget that each part-time employee counts as one, and also to include any trainee or part-time clinical assistant) must put this in writing
- carry out health surveillance of your employees where appropriate
- appoint a competent person (normally an employee) to help you devise and apply the protective steps identified as necessary by your risk assessment
- set up emergency procedures
- give employees information about health and safety matters

- co-operate on health and safety matters with other employers sharing your premises (eg the DHA or Health Board)
- make sure your employees have adequate health and safety training and are capable enough at their job to avoid risk
- give whatever health and safety information is needed by temporary staff to meet their needs.

These regulations also:

- place duties on all employees to follow health and safety instructions and report danger
- extend current health and safety law that requires you to consult employees' safety representatives and provide facilities for them.

All these general duties exist alongside the more specific ones laid down in other health and safety regulations, including the new ones described below. Of course, this does not mean you have to do things twice. For example, if you have done a risk assessment to comply with the Control of Substances Hazardous to Health (COSHH) Regulations, you need not repeat the exercise to comply with those new general management regulations.

Provision and use of work equipment

These regulations pull together and tidy up various laws governing equipment used at work. Instead of piecemeal legislation covering particular kinds of equipment in different industries, these:

- place general duties on all employers;
- list minimum requirements for work equipment, to deal with selected hazards that apply to all industries and sectors.

The regulations make explicit what is already provided for in current legislation or good practice. If you have well-chosen and well-maintained equipment you should not need to do any more. Guidance on the regulations reinforces this point. Although some older equipment may need to be upgraded to meet the minimum requirements, you have until 1997 to do this. You should not allow your practice to be bamboozled by local tradesmen who try to frighten you and your colleagues into employing them to undertake health and safety checks.

The general duties of these regulations require a practice to:

- take into account the working conditions and hazards in your surgery premises when choosing equipment
- ensure that your equipment is suitable for the use you intend to make of it and that it is properly maintained
- give adequate information, instruction and training.

Box 13.3: Definition of 'work equipment'

'Work equipment' is broadly defined to include everything from a hand tool, through machines of all kinds, to a complete plant such as an oil refinery. 'Use' includes starting, stopping, installing, dismantling, programming, setting, transporting, maintaining, servicing and cleaning.

Specific requirements cover:

- guarding of dangerous parts of machinery (replacing the existing law on this)
- maintenance arrangements
- dangers caused by equipment failure
- parts and materials at high or very low temperatures
- control systems and devices
- isolation of equipment from power sources
- physical stability of equipment
- lighting
- warnings and markings.

These Regulations implement an EC Directive aimed at the protection of workers. There are other Directives setting out the conditions that much new equipment must satisfy before it can be sold in EC member states. These are implemented in the UK by regulations made by the Department of Trade and Industry. Any equipment that satisfies these other Directives on standards should satisfy many of the specific requirements listed above.

Manual handling operations

These regulations replace patchy, old-fashioned and largely ineffective legislation with a modern ergonomic approach to the problem. They are important because the incorrect handling of loads causes many injuries, resulting in pain, time off work and even permanent disablement.

The regulations apply to any manual handling operations that may cause injury at work; these should have been identified by the risk assessment carried out under the general health and safety management regulations described above. They include not only the lifting of loads but also lowering, pushing, pulling, carrying or moving them, whether by hand or by other bodily force. Again, these Regulations are supported by general guidance.

There are health care activities where staff are at risk; an obvious example is nursing. You have to take three key steps:

- avoid hazardous manual handling operations where reasonably practicable
- assess adequately any hazardous operations that cannot be avoided
- reduce the risk of injury as far as practicable.

Health, safety and welfare at the workplace

These regulations tidy up existing legislation, replacing some 35 pieces of old law, including parts of the Factories Act 1961 and the Offices, Shops and Railway Premises Act 1963. They are much easier to understand, making it far clearer what is expected of employers. The regulations cover many aspects of health, safety and welfare in the workplace, setting general requirements in four broad areas.

Working environment
- temperature
- ventilation
- lighting, including emergency lighting
- room dimensions
- suitability of workstations.

Safety
- safe passage of pedestrians and vehicles (eg traffic routes must be wide enough and properly marked)
- windows and skylights (safe opening, closing and cleaning)
- transparent/translucent doors and partitions (use of safe material and marking)
- doors, gates and escalators (safety devices)
- floors (construction and maintenance, obstructions, and slipping and tripping hazards)
- falls from height
- falling objects (eg from cupboards or shelves).

Facilities
- toilets
- washing, eating and changing facilities
- clothing storage
- seating
- rest areas (and arrangements in them for non-smokers)
- rest facilities for pregnant women and nursing mothers.

Housekeeping
- maintenance of workplace, equipment and facilities
- cleanliness
- removal of waste materials.

You have to ensure that your surgery complies with the Regulations, but this does not have to be completed until 1996 for an existing surgery. Other people connected with your surgery premises (eg the owner of a building that is leased to one or more employers or self-employed people) also have to ensure that requirements falling within their control are satisfied. Again, these Regulations are supported by an approved code of practice.

Box 13.4: Definition of 'personal protective equipment'

This is all equipment designed to be worn or held to protect against a risk to health or safety. It includes most types of protective clothing and equipment such as eye, foot and head protection, safety harnesses, life jackets and high visibility clothing. There are some exceptions; for example, ordinary working clothes and uniforms (including clothes provided for food hygiene), those provided for road transport (eg crash helmets) and sports equipment.

Personal protective equipment

These regulations set out principles for selecting, providing, maintaining and using personal protective equipment.

Personal protective equipment (known as PPE) should be relied upon only as a last resort. Nevertheless, where risks are adequately controlled by other means, employers have a duty to provide suitable equipment, free of charge, for all employees exposed to those risks. Personal protective equipment is suitable only if it: is appropriate for the risks and the working conditions; takes account of your staff's needs and fits them properly; gives adequate protection; and is compatible with any other PPE they may wear.

You also have duties to:

- assess the risk and the PPE you intend to issue, to ensure that it is suitable
- maintain, clean and replace PPE
- provide storage for PPE when not being used
- ensure that PPE is properly used
- give training, information and instruction on its use.

All new PPE must comply with an EC Directive on design, certification and testing. This is implemented in the UK by Regulations made by the Department of Trade and Industry, but you are allowed to use PPE bought before the implementation of these regulations.

VDU Health and Safety regulations

Unlike the other Regulations outlined above, the Health and Safety (Display Screen Equipment) Regulations do not replace old legislation but cover a new area of work activity for the first time. Generally, working with VDUs is not a high-risk activity, but it can lead to muscular and other physical problems, eye fatigue and mental stress. Problems of this kind can be overcome by good ergonomic design of equipment, furniture, working environment and tasks performed.

The regulations apply to those VDUs where there is a 'user'; that is, an employee who habitually uses it as a significant part of normal work. They cover equipment used for the display of text, numbers and graphics regardless of the display process used.

The employer's duties include:

* assessing VDU workstations and reducing risk that are identified
* making sure that workstations satisfy minimum requirements set for the VDU itself, keyboard, desk and chair, working environment and task design, and software
* planning VDU work so that there are breaks or changes in activity
* providing information and training for VDU users.

VDU users are also entitled to appropriate eye and eyesight tests, and to special glasses if they are needed and normal ones cannot be used.

Again, these regulations are supported by detailed guidelines.

Further reading

The Health and Safety Executive publishes a comprehensive range of guides to the new regulations:

Management of health and safety at work. Approved code of practice. £5 ISBN 0 11 886330 4

Work equipment. £5 ISBN 0 11 886332 0

Manual handling. £5 ISBN 0 11 886335 5

Workplace health, safety and welfare. Approved code of practice. £5 ISBN 0 11 886333 9

Personal protective equipment at work. £5 ISBN 0 11 886334 7

Display screen equipment work. £5 ISBN 0 11 886331 2

These are all available from HMSO Bookshops and Agents or can be ordered from HMSO Publications Centre, PO Box 276, London SW8 5DT (mail, fax and telephone orders only):

General enquiries   071-873 0011
Telephone orders   071-873 9090
Fax orders   071-873 8200

The employees' responsibilities

Staff are required to take reasonable care for their own health and safety on the premises, and, for the safety of other users of the premises who may be affected by their actions, to co-operate with the employer in carrying out these duties.

Although the duties of employees apply 'while at work', it would be wise to assume that these apply throughout the time they remain on the premises. This is important because accidents can occur when staff are preparing tea or lunch in a staff rest room.

Staff must not interfere with or misuse any equipment provided for the purposes of health and safety, such as fire exits, fire extinguishers, and any warning notices. This includes any safety procedures applying to a kitchen, cloakroom or rest room.

How is the law enforced?

It is important to remember that the Health and Safety at Work Act is a criminal statute and the HSE an enforcement body. Failure to carry out any duty under the Act constitutes an offence and can lead to a prosecution, fine or imprisonment.

However, the HSE is firmly committed to persuasion. It has discretion to decide whether to prosecute and does so only after careful consideration of advice from the inspector. If a prosecution should arise, the courts would assess what is reasonably practicable in the light of available resources.

Each area of the country has its own inspectors, and one or more of these will be specifically concerned with health service premises, including GP surgeries. Each inspector has considerable powers and these are stated in his warrant of appointment. He may enter any premises to enforce this law, and does not need to seek permission before doing so. However, he can enter only at a 'reasonable time'.

In practice, notice is given of a visit and an inspector will telephone to arrange an appointment. Very rarely, 'surprise' inspections are made in response to a complaint from an employee or a user of the premises. Otherwise, the only reason why unannounced visits are made is that the inspector finds that he has some spare time available and includes a visit to

a small premises within his organized schedule of visits to larger estab-
lishments. Although these 'surprise' visits have caused anxiety, no offence is
intended and the inspector should not be suspected of harbouring an ulterior
motive.

An inspection

If there are five or more staff, the inspector will wish to see a statement of
safety policy and instructions on safety procedures. He will also want to see
the accident book.

The inspector will examine the electrical equipment. This should be in
good working order and there should be adequate maintenance arrangements. The toilet and washing facilities should be at least equal to those
required in offices. In particular, he will probably expect to find a supply of
hot and cold running water, and he may even propose elbow-operated taps
in all rooms used for examining and treating patients.

There are other matters, including the heating system, drug storage
arrangements, steam sterilizers, clinical waste disposal, and heating and
lighting standards, an inspector will also be concerned about.

When he has completed the inspection the inspector will normally raise
directly any improvements required with the person in administrative charge
of the surgery. If these matters are not of major importance he will just request
that they are carried out as soon as possible.

More serious matters could lead to a formal letter, or even a written notice
requiring them to be put right within a specified period of time – not less than
21 days. In these circumstances the inspector would also warn the staff of his
intention to serve a written notice.

In the most unlikely circumstances of there being a serious risk to health
and safety, which should never occur in a GP's surgery, the inspector can
issue a prohibition notice. Where there is a very serious risk, all work has to
stop immediately.

The accident book

The employer is obliged to keep an accident book, in which all notifiable
accidents and occurrences are recorded. This enables the employer to monitor
these and take action to prevent any recurrence. A record book is published
by the Health and Safety Executive (Record of Accidents, Dangerous Occurrences and Ill-Health Enquiries, F2509, HMSO). It is interesting to note that
any self-employed person is exempt from this reporting procedure; the GP
need not report any accident to himself.

An action list

1 A written statement of policy on health and safety should be issued to all staff, if there are five or more employees. This written statement can be included in the contracts of employment.
2 Keep an accident book and copies of form 2508, the accident report form.
3 Electrical equipment should be regularly maintained and serviced.
4 One member of the staff may be appointed as the 'safety officer'. The practice manager may be best able to take on this responsibility.
5 Any known hazards should be checked at regular intervals to see if improvements need to be made. Obvious examples include loose floor coverings, any building work, electrical plugs and equipment.
6 Patients and visitors should be warned by written notices of any hazards on the premises. This is particularly important if there are building works in progress.
7 The premises' lease of licence agreement should be reviewed. This should state who is responsible for maintaining and repairing the premises. If in doubt, contact the BMA local office.

14 Managing for Quality Care

Introduction

This last chapter is about quality. The most important driving force for quality of work comes from within, as each of us strives to carry out tasks as best we can. Leadership within a practice is crucial and the example and standard set by the practice manager is a key factor. Quality must start at the top, so that every member of the practice team can see what is expected of them. They should experience both the reward of knowing when they have done well and receive guidance when things have not gone as well as expected. However, there are also external measures and controls to be acknowledged and these include external complaints procedures and external quality standards – both of which deserve consideration.

Complaints and litigation

The prime responsibility that doctors and their staff have is, of course, to patients and there is a natural desire to provide the 'best' service they possibly can. However, they are also accountable in various ways to other bodies. Staff are accountable to their employers – the doctors; doctors are accountable to the Family Health Services Authority to abide by the terms and conditions of their contracts and doctors are also accountable to their registering body, the General Medical Council. These lines of accountability should not be seen as threats to independence or security, but as part of the system for maintaining the quality of work. The chances of anyone falling foul of them is small indeed but it is still worth thinking about the various relationships and how doctors and staff can remain on the right side of authorities.

There are a growing number of complaints about all parts of the health service. The reasons for this increase are obscure. In part it may be due to a more intense scrutiny of the activities of all the professions, eg lawyers, teachers and accountants, in relation to their self-regulation. It is also clearly affected by an increase in 'consumerism' stimulated by more emphasis on rights set out in Charters and less emphasis on responsibilities and, lastly, in part to an increased tendency for people in all walks of life to seek redress under the law.

The best safeguard is, of course, a constant attention to the quality of work. However, mistakes do happen, or appear to happen, and need to be properly attended to – every practice is familiar with situations where patients feel they are not getting the service to which they are entitled. Indeed most of us would feel that patients have every right to have high expectations of the service.

A person who is ill is vulnerable, more likely to feel threatened and become angry and someone who is acting on behalf of a patient tends to be more demanding for they view themselves as the 'champion' of the patient. Staff should recognize that this anger or these feelings may be directed at them even if they are not the appropriate target. In many cases, the victim is just lashing out and their anger is a symptom of anxiety. Dealing with such behaviour requires a considerable amount of professionalism. It is not well handled by getting angry oneself but needs understanding and tact. The practice manager has an important training role towards her staff in this area and a vital role in setting a personal example.

If a difficult situation arises at the receptionist's desk, the practice manager should be prepared to intervene and invite the patient into a private area so that neither the patient, staff or others in the building become concerned. In the same way, if a difficult matter arises on the telephone, the practice manager should take over and if unable to sort matters out invite the patient to come and see her to discuss the issue. In cases of disagreement between patients and the practice, it is difficult to strike the right balance between loyalty to the practice and loyalty to the patient, and whilst the old adage 'the customer is always right' should not be taken too literally, it is a useful generalization to bear in mind. It is worth noting that in the majority of cases where a patient is complaining they are not seeking redress but an assurance that such a problem will not arise again either for themselves or for others. It is often the experience of those dealing with formal complaints that many could have been settled by prompt and tactful action and, often, by an apology. Sometimes patients treated in such a way become the most loyal supporters of the practice, although there is always the danger that an apology will be seen as an admission of error whereas it may be an attempt to defuse a situation.

Staff rudeness must never be tolerated and the practice manager needs to exercise a very firm hand here. If a complaint is significant, the doctors should always be informed of the action taken and, if there is any likelihood of it going further, it is important to make careful notes at the time.

The Family Health Services Authority

Each individual doctor has a contract with the FHSA. He or she is not an employee, so the Authority is not responsible for any of the actions of any of the people within the practice. However, the doctor is bound by terms and conditions of service as set out in the 'Red Book'. Many of these are concerned with accessibility and availability and, for example, require doctors to be available to patients out of hours and surgeries to be open when they are said to be open. Others are related to payments made by the FHSA, for example, a practice obtaining financial support for their premises will be expected to provide premises of an acceptable standard. The practice manager will have a detailed knowledge of these and may need to remind staff of them from time to time.

A more difficult area is where a patient feels so aggrieved about the medical care given that they make a complaint to the FHSA that, for example, the doctor failed to make the correct diagnosis. The FHSA is not empowered to investigate such matters but often has an informal role in arbitrating, and many problems are settled in this way, particularly if the principle issue is a failure to understand caused by a breakdown in communication. The FHSA will have a formal role in issues of clinical care if the doctor has failed to put him or herself in a position to make a correct diagnosis by not visiting, not keeping proper records, not referring to the hospital or for investigation or not providing an appointment reasonably promptly – all of which are requirements of the terms and conditions of service. It can be seen that good evidence may be vital in securing a proper defence against such allegations. Written guidelines for staff about appointments, the way to deal with requests for visits, off duty arrangements and so on will help to establish what is the 'normal' procedure followed and well kept message books and appointment books will add support. Ensuring that notes are available to doctors whenever they see a patient is good practice and proper systems for dealing with reports and letters will not only provide high quality care but will also support proof of such care if every it is needed (*see also* page 208).

The General Medical Council

Doctors have to be registered with the General Medical Council in order to practice as a doctor within the National Health Service. The responsibilities of the Council are derived from this duty to keep the Register and, in pursuit of the quality of doctors' work, they set the standards for training and thus decide who may be entered on the Register. By promulgating ethical advice and advice on behaviour they give guidance to doctors on the Register as to how they should practice and, where a lapse from such standards occurs, they have the power to remove or suspend a doctor from the Register or to make conditions apply to the registration. Suspension or conditions of registration are also used where a doctor's fitness to practice is impaired by ill health or problems with drug or alcohol dependence. Patients often feel that they would like misdiagnosis to be enough to be considered as a reason for complaint to the GMC. However, unless the failure is so serious that the doctor could be removed from the Register, for that is at present the only sanction the GMC has been given by the Medical Act, the complaint will not be successful.

Civil litigation

Neither the FHSA nor the GMC are well equipped to deal with a potential failure of clinical standards of care, and it is only if a patient turns to civil litigation that redress for damage caused by a medical mistake can be obtained. This is a lengthy and expensive business. Patients may be put off taking this course of action if they are not legally aided and many may also be deterred by the wear and tear caused by the length of any proceedings. The wear and tear on doctors is also considerable and can produce severe anxiety and exhaustion even when the complaint is not upheld. Doctors have professional indemnity insurance so that the financial penalty of defending themselves is not in itself a burden. For the practice manager, the provision of high standards of quality is the best way she can support both her patients and her employers.

Setting quality standards

The concept of setting quality standards which are recognized with an external award has been around in industry for many years. The most well-known is the kite mark on manufactured products that assures the customer that certain production and safety standards have been achieved. There are obvious benefits to companies providing a service or manufacturing a product who have this type of recognition.

The recent introduction of the Patient's Charter has highlighted the need for accountability in general practice. The general practitioner is no longer considered to be on a pedestal, and is more likely to be challenged by patients about their accessibility and the range of services they receive. This change in patient attitude demands an equal change in general practice. Many people working within the health service would welcome some kind of external award, however, presently, the main awards are those available to industry, although the King's Fund has a quality package aimed at primary health care teams.

There are distinct advantages in applying for an external award:

- it gives the whole practice team a corporate aim and in doing so clarifies the necessary standards to be set and then maintained;
- it may attract new patients;
- the practice team must work together to review the range of services on offer and match these to the patients' needs.

Like any initiative to improve quality, there are time and money costs to be considered. A complete practice review will need to have resources devoted to it and will need a suitable person with enough authority to tackle the more difficult areas and sufficient enthusiasm to maintain the momentum to lead it. This type of exercise will only look at operational standards and does not include any aspects of clinical care – these must be dealt with via the more usual channels of protocols and clinical audits from medical records.

If a practice does detail the standards of service a patient can reasonably expect, for example, that all patients requesting urgent appointments will be offered one on the same day, then it must introduce systems to maintain them. Should the practice fail to meet its own standards then the number of complaints may increase. The first priority to improve quality could be to introduce a complaints procedure that all staff are trained to observe.

It is important that any new standards are realistic and attainable, otherwise the exercise is pointless and the team will become demoralized. It is acceptable to modify a Practice Charter and work steadily towards higher standards – this is better than no Charter at all.

Charter Mark Scheme

This award was introduced in 1991 to recognize excellence in the delivery of public services. In 1993 there were 100 awards available and all groups within the NHS were eligible to apply, including general practice.

The criteria for judging in 1993 were:

- standards;
- information and openness;
- choice and consultation;
- courtesy and helpfulness;
- putting things right;
- value for money;
- customer satisfaction;
- measurable improvements in the quality of service over the last two or more years;
- plans to introduce, or have underway, at least one innovative enhancement to services without any additional cost to the taxpayer or consumer.

There is an explanatory booklet, *The Charter Mark Scheme* which is available from:

> Citizens' Charter Unit,
> Office of Public Service and Science,
> Cabinet Office,
> Horse Guards Road,
> London SW1P 3AL

The booklet gives case studies and examples to explain how some of the award winning organizations have prepared for their application. Any practice wishing to apply should contact their FHSA to obtain a current copy of the booklet and an application form.

BS5750 – BSI quality assurance

The British Standard Institute is responsible for the kite mark which appears on some manufactured goods, and it also runs a certification and assessment service aimed at commerce. The BS5750 is the national standard for quality management systems and was first published in 1979. Over the last few years it has been extended to more service-based industries and organizations. In itself the standard is quite general and encompasses 20 requirements which a company should follow to ensure a quality of service or product. It concentrates on the appropriateness of service in relation to the consumer's needs.

To achieve approval for BS5750 the practice must first complete a document which details each system in operation to deliver the various services. When the application has been submitted an assessment team will visit the practice to see the systems working and to check that the theory matches actual practice. Part of the check is to ensure that the practice has sufficient resources to meet the requirements. The size of the team will vary in accordance with the organization to be assessed and the complexity of the application. If the organization is successfully registered there will be continuing visits to ensure that the quality is being maintained. In common with other major quality initiatives, BS5750 will only be successful if all staff are involved in the planning and preparation of the application, and effectively trained in all aspects of their role within the organization.

To obtain further information about BS5750 for general practice contact:

> Health Services Sector,
> BSI Quality Assurance,
> PO Box, 375,
> Milton Keynes MK14 6LL

The King's Fund

The King's Fund in conjunction with other professional and consumer groups, has developed a method of assessing quality within primary health care teams called The King's Fund Organizational Audit.

There are three stages:

1   The practice introduces the organizational standards and criteria with the help of the King's Fund staff who have been designated to the project.

The whole process takes roughly nine months and includes all staff, often divided into small working parties to review a particular aspect of the practice. The team then assesses how well it is conforming to the agreed standards.

2   The practice is the subject of a two day survey by an independent team.
3   At the end of the survey the practice receives instant verbal feedback, followed by a written report.

For more information contact:

> Primary Health Care Programme,
> King's Fund Organizational Audit,
> 2 Palace Court,
> London W2 4HS

As previously mentioned, there is a financial cost to practices wishing to embark on a recognized standard, these currently stand at approximately £2600 for the BS5750 and £6500 for the King's Fund Organizational Audit.

There are benefits to any practice wishing to undertake a complete review of their services, not least of which is the opportunity to involve all the staff in a programme that results in common aims and objectives. By using staff to examine an area of the practice that they may not be familiar with is an ideal way to broaden their understanding of the way the whole practice works, and to be more aware of the needs of other members of the team.

Conclusion

If this book has been read from cover to cover one could be forgiven for believing that managing a practice is an almost impossible task. The range of technical and personal skills seem endless, probably only found in some kind of super-being. The reality is slightly different – the practice manager needs to maximize the skills of the team and it is not necessary to have them all personally.

There are a few recurrent themes that any practice manager should treat as personal priorities – setting high standards, training the team to meet them and open channels of communication between the whole practice team. The practice manager also has another obligation, and that is to train people for the future and enable them to become involved in the management role and, also, to continue a programme of personal development to prepare for all the challenges that lie ahead. This can be on a formal basis, for example, to train a deputy to take over in the fullness of time, or by encouraging each individual to fulfil their own potential. Staff always respond to additional responsibility, it enhances their perceived value to the practice and increases their self-esteem and confidence.

The practice manager's most effective personal skill is self-analysis, to be completely honest about the things that he or she does well or badly. The most successful technique is to concentrate on one's strengths and look for ways to utilize the strengths of others within the team to minimize one's weaknesses. The practice manager therefore needs to know the staff as individuals as well as employees.

Fortunately there are an increasing number of similarities between managing a practice and management in industry and commerce, and this has opened up a whole range of training opportunities for managers within the health service. There are a number of courses and seminars on all aspects of management that each manager should consider for their own development. It could be a new skill, like wordprocessing, or updating an existing skill, like interviewing techniques. The temptation is to think 'that won't apply to the NHS' when a course is advertised, but motivating a workforce demands the same range of skills whether it is a chocolate factory or a GP practice. In industry the management team receive training in leadership, communications, appraisals, effective meetings and negotiation skills, to name just a few. They all have an application for today's practice manager. Most colleges can offer a course, or will be willing to tailor make one if a group of managers agree the topics and are willing to attend. There are also numerous management consultants testing the general practice market. Before agreeing to use a consultancy group for a course or an away day it is wise to ask them for a list of people for whom they have done work, and then telephone for references. Consultancy companies are not cheap, and a little background effort could avoid a costly mistake. If the training you need is not readily available contact the FHSA to see if it can be arranged, because if you are interested the chances are that other managers will also be keen to attend.

General practice is a business that demands a professional approach from every member of the team, the practice manager's duty is to set an example and to help others to achieve the same high standards.

Index